DESIGNING and BUILDING your own PROFESSIONAL OFFICE

Murray Schwartz, D.D.S.
Foreword by Mark S. Masch, M.D.

Medical Economics Company
Book Division
Oradell, New Jersey 07649

Library of Congress Cataloging in Publication Data

Schwartz, Murray.
    Designing and building your own professional office.

    Includes index.
        1. Medical offices—Planning.   2. Medical offices—
Design and construction.   I. Title.
R728.S42   610'.68'2   80-27712
ISBN 0-87489-228-7

Design by Elaine Kilcullen

ISBN 0-87489-228-7

Medical Economics Company Inc.
Oradell, New Jersey 07649

Printed in the United States of America

First Printing   July, 1981
Second Printing   July, 1982

With love to Marcia,
who started the whole idea,
and to Esther, Danny, and Jonathan

CONTENTS

FOREWORD

Every morning was the same. The thought of going into work was depressing. My office was dingy and cramped; the traffic pattern defied all attempts at efficiency. If it depressed *me,* what was it doing to my patients? I decided to move.

First, I had to decide whether to deal with another landlord or build my own office. I chose to build. That saddled me with the tasks of finding partners to share the financial load; retaining lawyers to draw up contracts, partnership arrangements, and bills of sale; and shopping for mortgage money. Compared to the rest, that was the easy part.

Talking with other doctors who had built their own offices was enlightening. The conversations followed a similar pattern. At first, they all seemed content with their accomplishments, admitting only an occasional ``I-should-have-done-this-instead-of-that.'' The more we talked, the more this-instead-of-thats cropped up. It usually took less than five minutes for the truth to out. The experience was a ``Never, never again'' horror. How could I avoid their mistakes? Simple: I would be different, I would rely on the experts to put my building together. Each would be allowed to do his own thing. Not so simple:

For starters, I didn't have the unlimited funds it takes to hire an unlimited array of experts. Besides, I didn't even know who the experts were, or where to find them. I ended up making the decisions on site layout, parking, building design, office design, structural materials, and more. I had to do a lot of research.

I had to learn about heating, air conditioning, insulation, electrical outlets, plumbing, and more. I had to deal with the *experts* in these fields.

I learned that some were not so expert; that their concerns were not always consistent with my own best interests. I spent whole days, then weeks and months on my building. It took time, and then more time. I learned and I compromised. Particularly, I learned to compromise.

Worst of all was the feeling of being stranded, alone in a jungle, somehow having to survive and reach safety without a guide. I reached a real understanding of the emotional costs of all those conversational this-instead-of-thats. And only when my building was finished and my office running smoothly did I feel prepared to start my own project. Would I do it again? I'll put it this way:

Murray Schwartz also built his own office. Before, during, and after, he gleaned practical know-how from physicians, dentists, and other professionals who had done it, from dozens of experts, and from scores of publications. He put it all into a coherent, logical framework that he calls *Designing and Building Your Own Professional Office.* It doesn't pretend to solve all the problems of deciding where and how to move or build. It does teach you the questions to ask; and how you resolve those questions will put your personal stamp on your project. But it will also do much more.

With this book you won't be alone in the jungle. It will help sustain you through the trials ahead; it will be your steadfast guide and companion.

For all that, the book is guilty of an unforgivable fault. It was written after my building was completed. But as for my next building. . .

Mark S. Masch, M.D.
Upper Nyack, NY

PREFACE

"It took us a year after we moved in to get all the bugs out. Some of the details I just never thought of, and now it's too late and expensive to do anything about them."

"That damn architect never told me it was going to cost this much and take this long."

"I thought I'd save a few bucks by contracting it myself. What a mistake!"

You've probably heard doctors make complaints like these about their experiences in establishing new offices. But it doesn't have to be that way. The creation of a new office that is efficient, attractive, comfortable, and affordable should not be a hit-or-miss affair.

There are sound strategies that have worked for others; they will work for you, too, once you learn them. You may be a physician, dentist, or other health professional. You may have just completed your training and are opening your first office. You may be an established practitioner seeking new quarters. Whatever your situation, this book can be your guide.

Doctors' offices differ from one another in many ways: by specialty, equipment, number of doctors and assistants, and volume of patients. Yet, despite these differences, the new-office needs of most health professionals are surprisingly alike in the details and the problems to be considered.

Usually, doctors are inadequately prepared for these problems, and you're, no doubt, no exception. Almost certainly, the curriculum in your professional school did not provide you with more than a rudimentary idea of how an office is created. Even if you've practiced for years you may not be sure of the best way to proceed.

There are professionals in this field—architects, space planners, interior designers, practice-management consultants, supply houses, and builders—who are eager to do the job for you for a fee, but each of them views the project from his own point of view rather than from that of the doctor.

This book, written from the doctor's viewpoint, describes for you many of the elements involved in buying, building, or leasing your new office. It gives you a good idea of what is in store for you.

It suggests guidelines for obtaining the right amount of space and for controlling the sequence of events, for choosing an architect, for evaluating a floor plan, and for designing mechanical systems. It can make you knowledgeable enough to spot many of the errors that can creep into every construction project. These errors, if not corrected promptly, lead to expensive delays later when their correction is more difficult.

Even more important, the book offers many of the right questions to ask during the planning stages to avoid costly omissions. Wherever possible, it provides numbers: estimates of costs, sizes of important items, and frequently used rules of thumb.

How did I get involved in writing this book? I'm a periodontist and a professor of dentistry who, with my partner, practice in our own newly renovated building. It was during our construction that I realized how helpful this kind of book could be to every doctor who needed a new office.

With some prior knowledge, and with my own firsthand experience in the creation of our office, I felt that I had enough material to start this project. Further research and communications with other doctors and with specialists in the office-construction field provided additional information. My goal is to pass along to you what I have learned.

I recognize that there is a large and growing number of women in all of the professions, but you'll find that I've used masculine pronouns when alluding to doctors, architects, and builders. Until someone invents some satisfactory terms, this is the only way I know to refer to these individuals without exceptionally awkward sentences.

PUBLISHER'S NOTES

What you'll find here in Murray Schwartz's book are specific guidelines to help you every step of the way to a new office: from making the basic choice between renting, subleasing, renovating, buying, or building, right through to moving in and organizing office maintenance.

The guidelines go into great detail, but their specific nature doesn't mean that they're appropriate for only one kind of office. Dr. Schwartz has made them universally applicable. They're practical directions for you to follow, no matter who your architect is, how large your office must be, what equipment you need, whatever your field or specialty happens to be.

Nor are the plans shown in the book intended to be specific models for you to use. Rather, they're examples of principles you should follow.

The usefulness of the book for you lies in its being written from your point of view. It details what you have to look out for; it gives primary importance to *your* interests.

Dr. Schwartz went through the process of renovating and adding an extension to an older building. In planning the construction for his office, and then, to a greater extent, in writing this book, Dr. Schwartz consulted with dozens of physicians and dentists who had planned the construction, furnishing, and equipping of new offices. His key question to all of them was: "Now that you've been through it all, what do you know now that you wish you knew before you started?" This book is the distillation of the answers and of his actual experience in seeing his own office evolve from preliminary plans to working reality.

Dr. Schwartz, clinical professor and director of undergraduate periodontics at Columbia University School of Dental and Oral Surgery, practices in Nyack, N.Y. The photographs and line drawings in the book are his own.

Mark S. Masch, M.D., who wrote the Foreword, practices internal medicine in the office he built in Upper Nyack, N.Y.

ACKNOWLEDG-
MENTS

I needed the assistance and cooperation of outstanding people to write this book.

William Eli Kohn, A.I.A., graciously reviewed the entire manuscript, correcting errors, filling gaps, and adding details.

My partner, Dr. Michael B. Savin, provided important comments on many of the subjects. His recollections of our problems in office construction were valuable supplements to my own. Dr. Robert Gottsegen's aid and encouragement helped to get the project started. Dr. Bernard Moskow offered much-needed guidance about photographic problems.

Manuel S. Emanuel, A.I.C.P., an urban planner, skillfully led me through the maze of zoning laws and other land-use regulations. Murray S. Korn, C.P.A., and Harris L. Markhoff, LL.B., added to my understanding of many accounting and legal details.

Many doctors, medical and dental, shared with me their triumphs and traumas in office creation.

Mrs. E. Pearl Krebs spent countless hours typing draft after draft of the manuscript.

To all of you I offer my thanks for your help and advice. Any errors or omissions, which I hope are few, are my sole responsibility.

M.S.

HOW TO USE THIS BOOK

Start with three basic principles:

Get involved! Be part of the planning process at every stage. Don't expect any adviser to do it for you. You can make intelligent choices only if you're fully aware of what is going on.

Don't try to do it all yourself! Unless you're a trained architect or builder you'll probably lose more than you'll gain by trying to design and contract the office entirely on your own. Get professional help.

Look twice before you leap! The most important and expensive decisions are the very first ones. Don't commit yourself to anything until you've read the appropriate sections of this book.

You'll get the most from the book if you first go through it rapidly to get an idea of how the office creation process works. Read the first section (Chapters 1 to 4) carefully. Work out the possibilities for yourself about whether to lease, buy, or build.

Next, decide what kind of advisers you'll need and how to find them. Then find them before you do anything else. You should have your business consultant or architect or space planner, for example, *before* you go looking for space to rent or land to buy.

Prior to your meetings with an architect, designer, or any other adviser, reread the parts of the book dealing with the subjects to be discussed. Make your own list of items to cover. The wish lists and checklists in the book suggest the questions to ask. The more knowledgeable you are, the more you'll get from these specialists.

When construction begins, keep the book with you when you visit the building site or the rented space that is to be altered. If the new office is distant from where you now work, you'll need to be especially well-prepared, since every visit to the job must be a fruitful one.

The book is arranged in the sequence likely to be followed if you lease office space or if you decide to build a professional office building with a total area not exceeding about 10,000 square feet. If you lease space, just omit the parts dealing with building construction and concentrate on those covering planning and construction in the office itself. These subjects are virtually the same whether you're building or renting.

Note that the book doesn't deal with deciding on a locality in which to practice. How to make such a decision is a separate topic, amply covered in books on starting a practice or on practice management.

The cost estimates are those of 1980. In our inflationary economy, you should figure on at least 10 to 12 percent annual increases in prices. Also, the costs mentioned are those in the New York metropolitan area. Elsewhere in the country, they will differ.

Good luck!

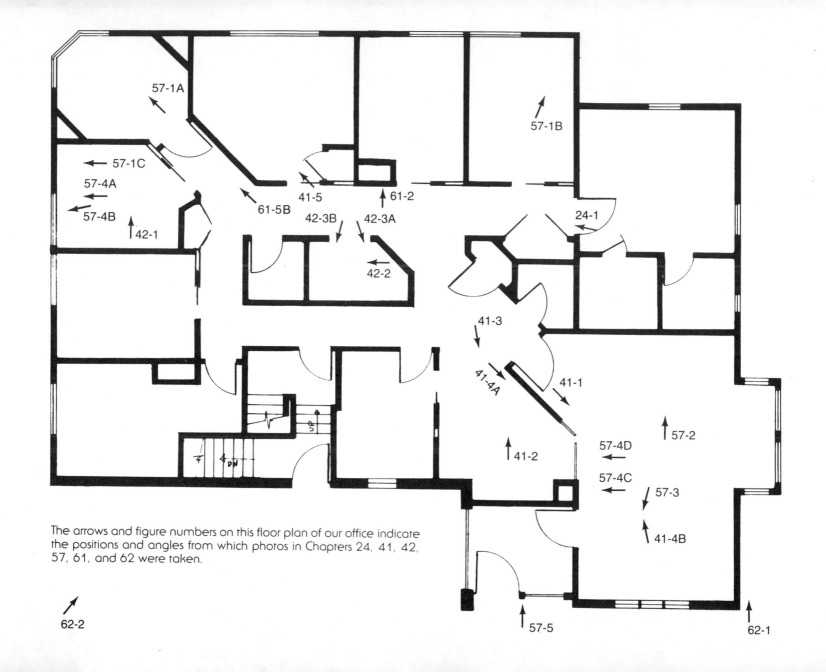

The arrows and figure numbers on this floor plan of our office indicate the positions and angles from which photos in Chapters 24, 41, 42, 57, 61, and 62 were taken.

I
GETTING STARTED

1
FIRST STEPS

Now that you've decided that a new office is in your future, you're probably wondering, "What should I do first?" In this chapter and in the rest of this section, you'll find ideas about how to begin and what your options are.

How much space do I need? More than you think! According to management consultants, doctors often decide on office suites before giving enough thought to how much room their practices require.

Here's a way to start estimating your space needs: List every room that you'd like to have, with its optimum size. This is the earliest version of the wish list that you'll need later. Right now, rough guesses will do. Table 1-1 is a sample list. You may want to omit some rooms and add others. Let me warn you now that three areas where space needs are most often badly underestimated are the business office, hallways, and storage.

The bottom line of Table 1-1 may surprise you if you've judged your needs correctly. Cost factors may force you to reduce some of the estimates later, but begin with optimum sizes. Once you have an estimate of your new office size, you'll be able to speak with more assurance to the experts you consult.

How much time will it take? More than you think! You're going to invest a lot of money in this office. Give yourself the chance to do it right.

Following are some approximations of the time it will take from the point at which you find a specific rental space or building site until you move in (these estimates include the time necessary for lease or purchase negotiations, planning, design, bidding, contracts, and the actual construction, decorating, and installations):

☐ leased or condominium space in an existing building: three to nine months;
☐ renovation of an old building: six to 18 months; and
☐ new building (your own): 12 to 24 months.

Note that these are my guesses of the time you'll need *after* you find the right spot. Finding it could take a day or a year or more.

If you're thinking of building, for example, start looking for an architect and assembling your team approximately two years before you hope to move in.

Think I'm being overly pessimistic? Maybe. But you'll find it much more comfortable to move when it suits *you* than to be forced out of your present office and into a half-finished suite.

How much will it cost? It depends. New-construction costs in my part of the country in mid-1980 were about $65 to $90 per square foot for a new small (up to 10,000 square feet) professional office building. Interior-construction costs in an existing building vary, depending on the amount and complexity of work to be done, but they are in the $20 to $40 per-square-foot range. The costs of equipment, furniture, and decorating are impossible to estimate because doctors' needs are so different. For furniture, floor covering, and wall covering, $10 to $12 per square foot is a rock-bottom figure.

Visit the offices of other doctors. You'll get ideas from each one about what to include and/or what to avoid in yours. Take a camera with you. Most doctors and their staffs will be flattered that you want to visit and take pictures. The photos will eliminate the need for excessive note-taking. Use 35mm or Polaroid fast color film. This will permit you to take most of your shots without distracting flashes, and you'll have a record of good and bad color schemes. But take along an electronic flash just in case.

You'll get some interesting responses if you ask each doctor, "What would you do differently if you were going to set up this office all over again?"

If you now have an office, this is the time to scrutinize everything about it. As you do so, note what you would like to retain or change. Prepare an inventory of which furniture and equipment is to be kept.

Your move to a new office is the ideal time to change any office systems that have outlived their usefulness. Review your record keeping, handling of correspondence, processing of insurance forms, billing, inventory control, instrument sterilization, and communication systems. If you have an office-procedure manual (and you should!), this will be the time to revise it.

It pays to think seriously about all of these points at a very early stage. Some of the changes you'll want will require special equipment or space that will have to be provided for in the plans.

TABLE 1-1

Estimating Office Space Needs

	Size desired	Sq. ft. needed per room	Number of such rooms	Total sq. ft. needed
Reception room	————	————	————	————
Business office	————	————	————	————
Private office	————	————	————	————
Exam/ treatment rooms	————	————	————	————
Laboratory	————	————	————	————
Staff lounge	————	————	————	————
Lavatory	————	————	————	————
Sterilization area	————	————	————	————
Storage and central supply	————	————	————	————
————	————	————	————	————
————	————	————	————	————

Total space needed for rooms and storage ———— sq. ft.

Add 25% (space needed for hallways, columns, walls, utility room, stairs, vestibule) + ———— sq. ft.

Total space requirement ———— sq. ft.

2
THE CHOICES: RENT, BUY, OR BUILD

There are many ways to establish an office. In this chapter, I list most of the possibilities with advantages and disadvantages of each. (Parts II and III discuss how to proceed after you've made your choice.) As you relate my comments to your own situation, keep these points in mind:

1. If you are just starting out in practice, flexibility will be one of your most important concerns. You'll probably want to lease space rather than buy or build. But you won't want to get involved with a long-term lease since your space needs may change.

2. Some of the choices mentioned won't be available when and where you want them. You may decide that it would be best for you to have your own professional office building. But if no suitable site is available, or if the zoning in the area prohibits such construction, you just can't do it.

3. If building your own office building appeals to you and adequate rental space is also available, you may be puzzled about how to compare the monetary risks and benefits involved in the two choices. The best approach is to have a professional business consultant or a competent real-estate specialist and a tax consultant do an analysis for you. Such studies are discussed in Chapter 12. If done properly, the analysis should give you a realistic idea of whether a new building would be a sound investment.

The advantages and disadvantages listed here are generalizations. You must carefully evaluate each of these considerations in the light of your specific circumstances.

LEASING UNFINISHED SPACE

Advantages:

1. Flexibility. You're free to leave at the end of the lease. A well-drawn lease offers an option for renewal, which permits you to stay if you wish.

2. The building's operating and maintenance problems are the landlord's responsibilities, not yours.

3. Large amounts of capital are not needed, except for equipping and furnishing your own office.

4. Less time is needed to plan, construct, and finish the office than what's required with construction of a new building.

5. The presence of other doctors in the building provides sources of referrals and exchanges of ideas.

6. The owners usually provide the service personnel needed for maintenance of your office (cleaning, floor waxing, painting, repairs).

7. You're not concerned with keeping the building fully occupied. You use your time as a doctor, not as a landlord.

Disadvantages:

1. No buildup of equity or inflation hedge is available.

2. You have no control over other tenants in the building (unless this is specified in the lease)—for example, whether other doctors in your specialty may also lease space in the building.

3. You have no direct control over the operation and the maintenance of the building.

4. There is no tax-sheltering benefit from the building's depreciation.

5. Rents increase with time at or above the rate of inflation. Landlords often demand steep increases at lease-renewal time, knowing that it would be more expensive for the doctor to move to other quarters than to pay the increased rent. Escalator clauses are frequently written in leases as a response to inflation.

6. Part of your initial investment, such as electrical and plumbing installations and some built-in cabinetwork, may not be recoverable when you decide to move out.

LEASING SPACE IN A HOSPITAL-OWNED BUILDING

In many communities, local hospitals have medical office buildings on their own grounds and lease space to staff doctors. Such arrangements have their own separate benefits and problems.

Advantages:

1. Seriously ill patients can be seen more frequently.
2. Substantial time is saved in travel to and from doctor's office and hospital. Doctor can see more patients per day.
3. Doctors in other specialties are available for ease of referral.
4. There is access to hospital's specialized services, pharmacy, and cafeteria.
5. Patient's travel time for hospital services is reduced.
6. You have less driving in bad weather.
7. The hospital's switchboard is available as answering service.

Disadvantages:

1. Rents may be higher than in nonhospital office buildings, especially if fireproof construction is required.
2. Tenants are likely to be more under hospital's control than doctors with offices away from hospital.
3. There is competition with services offered by hospital; lab and X-ray workups may be prohibited.
4. If a national health program is administered through hospitals, doctors in hospital-owned buildings may be the first to feel its effects.

SUBLEASING FURNISHED AND EQUIPPED SPACE

This is not likely to be your choice for your primary office, but it can be a convenient way to have a second office with minimal investment.

Advantages:

1. Maximum flexibility. You can usually leave with relatively short notice.
2. There's minimal investment. Small or no capital investment is needed for leasehold improvements, such as electrical work, plumbing, and cabinetry, or for expensive equipment.

3. You're not concerned with operating or maintenance problems in the building or in the office.

4. No construction delays of any kind are involved. You can sometimes begin work in the office on the same day you sign a lease agreement.

5. Rent is usually in proportion to amount of time the office is used.

6. Other doctors who have offices in the same building may be sources of referrals and consultation.

Disadvantages:

1. You have no control over the activities of other doctors who may use the same office.

2. Office layout may be a compromise.

3. As your practice expands, the office may not be available to you more hours per week.

4. Assistants working for other doctors may have personalities that you would consider inappropriate for office personnel.

5. You have no control over building operation.

6. You have no buildup of equity.

7. There's no tax shelter.

BUYING AN OFFICE CONDOMINIUM

This concept has become popular because it combines some of the attractive features of both rented space and custom new construction. The office unit is owned outright by the doctor, while the common areas—halls, elevators, lobby—are owned jointly with the other office occupants.

Advantages:

1. Your equity builds as the mortgage is amortized.

2. Tax shelter is available through depreciation.

3. Building operation and maintenance are handled by professionals.

4. Less capital outlay is involved than would be the case if you were owner of an entire building.

5. Sale is likely to be easier than having to sell an entire building.

6. Financing can be arranged separately for each office unit according to the owner's needs.

7. There is a possibility of income upon retirement. You may retain ownership of the office unit even after selling your practice. You may rent the office to the new doctor.

8. You have an inflation hedge. The value of the building increases with inflation. Mortgage payments remain constant, except with a variable-rate mortgage. (Mortgages are discussed in Chapter 18.)

Disadvantages:

1. You have less flexibility than you'd have with leasing, since a buyer or tenant must be found for your office if you choose to move. Meanwhile, you remain liable for regular payments of mortgage, taxes, and maintenance.

2. You have less control over building design and construction than if you were an owner of the entire structure.

3. You must abide by decisions of the building's management committee regarding the common areas, such as landscaping, hallway maintenance, operating costs.

4. You have little control over other occupants of the building.

5. If some owners default on mortgage payments, bank may take over their suites. New owners, to whom bank sells the space, may have an adverse effect upon the image of the building.

6. Invested capital earns no interest.

RENOVATING AN OLD BUILDING

Advantages:

1. Property is likely to be available at low cost.

2. Possibility exists of construction costs lower than costs of new construction, especially if room layout is suitable.

3. Minimal site improvement may be necessary. Landscaping has usually been done.

4. Part of the building may be suitable for conversion into additional offices or apartments.

5. Building's exterior may have favorable architectural features too expensive for new construction.

6. Special features may be present (such as the classic marble fireplace in our renovated building).

7. Build-up of equity occurs.

8. Inflation hedge exists.

9. Depreciation provides partial tax shelter.

10. Renovated older building may offer space at 30 to 40 percent lower cost than new construction.

11. Tax law (Revenue Act of 1978) offers tax credits for rehabilitation of old buildings under certain circumstances.

12. If your alterations result in energy conservation, you may be eligible for additional tax credit.

Disadvantages:

1. Existing room layout may be unsuitable and expensive to change.

2. Builders may be reluctant to offer firm bids for the job due to lack of detailed information about the original construction. For the same reason, some banks may be unwilling to lend maximum percentage of projected costs.

3. Utilities will often be inadequate and require replacement.

4. Maintenance and operating costs are likely to be higher than what can be expected in a newly constructed building.

5. Existing insulation may be inadequate.

6. Zoning change may be required to permit professional offices.

7. Possibility exists of neighborhood change.

8. Little flexibility. Resale may be difficult.

ENLARGING AND RENOVATING YOUR PRESENT OFFICE

Advantages:

1. Move to a new location is unnecessary.

2. Patients are acquainted with the location.

3. Construction and installations proceed under your constant supervision.

4. Renovating is usually less costly than a move to a new office.

Disadvantages:

1. Disruptions of your practice are likely for extended periods due to noise, dust, shut-offs of utilities, and need for moving equipment and furniture.

2. Strained relations may develop with nearby tenants because of the noise and dirt of construction.

3. The enlarged space may still be a compromise with what you really need.

4. Lease will have to be renegotiated, probably with a sharp rent increase.

BUYING A HOME-OFFICE COMBINATION

Advantages:

1. Build-up of equity occurs as mortgage is amortized.

2. Inflation hedge is available as value increases and mortgage payments remain constant.

3. Depreciation provides a partial tax shelter. Some of your household expenses become tax-deductible.

4. No daily commuting time or expense is needed.

5. You are likely to get many walk-in patients from the community.

6. It may be useful as a second office when your primary practice does not require your full-time attention.

Disadvantages:

If you are thinking of a home-office combination, *be careful*. In the opinion of many practice-management experts, this is not usually the best choice for a professional needing new office space, despite some initial apparent advantages. Only if the local zoning laws are permissive and the price of the property is exceptionally favorable should you consider the idea. These are some of the potential problems:

1. The home-office reduces your flexibility if you wish to move: If you hope to sell the building as a home-office combination you'll have to find another practitioner with virtually the same home and office needs. Local zoning may not permit use of the office by a doctor who is not also living in the house.

2. Zoning and building codes may prevent enlargement of the office or taking in an associate. Neighbors may oppose a zoning variance permitting a

larger office because of the likelihood of increased traffic in the neighborhood.

3. Even if permitted by zoning laws, it may be awkward to take in an associate later because the new doctor can never be truly equal while you live in the building. Also, your disability or death could present difficult problems in the transfer of the practice.

4. There will be a tendency for neighbors to impose on your free time for "emergency" services because you are just a few steps from your office.

5. It will require special efforts by you to avoid becoming isolated from your fellow doctors if this is your only office. Solo doctors in home-office combinations frequently have less exposure to new ideas than do their colleagues in other office environments.

6. It may be difficult to avoid family concerns during office hours. Unexpected intrusions by spouse, children, and pets may disrupt office routines.

BUILDING OR BUYING A SINGLE OFFICE BUILDING

Advantages:

1. The building is built according to your own needs and desires.

2. Provision for future expansion may be made.

3. You have no obligation either to a landlord or to a tenant. Only you and your partners in practice, if any, need to be satisfied.

4. Buildup of equity occurs as mortgage is amortized.

5. The building serves as an inflation hedge as its value increases, assuming location has been properly chosen.

6. Adequate return on initial investment is possible, if planned properly.

7. Building can provide office space at a net annual cost no greater than a leased suite.

8. Income-tax shelter is available through depreciation.

9. Some communities reduce real-estate taxes for a number of years to encourage new construction. In New York State, for example, towns and villages have the option of reducing taxes on new commercial buildings for a 10-year period after construction. This can mean savings of thousands of dollars.

10. High degree of satisfaction of doctor and staff.

Disadvantages:

1. Large cash outlay is required. Cost overruns are frequent in construction, requiring greater cash investment than planned.

2. Future sale may be difficult if the neighborhood deteriorates, if local zoning limits the type of use of the property, or if the later availability of ample rental space nearby limits the number of possible buyers.

3. Future sale will depend on finding a buyer with needs similar to yours.

4. The building's operation and maintenance are your responsibility.

5. Your practice may outgrow the building, requiring a major addition that may not be feasible; flexibility is severely limited.

6. Small buildings may have higher construction costs per square foot compared with larger structures.

7. You lose interest on invested capital.

8. More time is needed for construction than for preparing a rented suite for occupancy.

BUILDING OR BUYING A MULTIOFFICE BUILDING

Advantages:

1. Build-up of equity occurs as mortgage is amortized.

2. Your own office can be built exactly as you wish, with an ultimate square foot cost possibly no greater than rented space.

3. Inflation hedge develops as property value increases and mortgage payments remain constant.

4. Tax shelter exists through depreciation.

5. Adequate return on initial cash investment is possible if building is properly planned (positive cash flow).

6. If you have partners, your initial outlay is proportionately reduced.

7. Presence of partners can simplify sale at your retirement or death.

8. Real-estate-tax abatement may be available to encourage new construction in the area.

9. If you are the one who organizes and directs the project, your own cash investment may be reduced, or you may be rewarded in other ways.

Disadvantages:

1. Major cash outlay is needed.

2. If building is not fully rented there is a danger of expenses exceeding income (negative cash flow).

3. Cost overruns in construction can require such a large cash outlay that, even if building is fully rented, income may be insufficient to provide an adequate return on your investment. However, much of initial investment may be recovered by tax-sheltering effect of depreciation.

4. You—and partners, if any—have responsibility for operation and maintenance of the building, including the negotiation of leases with tenants and arranging for construction within their suites, or you'll have to pay for professional management. You'll have to cope with tenants' complaints.

5. Future construction of other office buildings nearby may create strong competition for tenants, especially if local hospital erects its own office building.

6. Danger exists of disagreements among partners and/or their spouses over some aspects of the project (see Chapter 13).

7. You suffer loss of interest on capital invested.

8. Much more time is needed for construction than for preparing a rented suite for occupancy.

9. Possibility exists that an unexpected change in your practice might result in a need for more space that would not be available. In effect, you could be locked into inadequate space in your own building.

BUILDING A MULTIOFFICE BUILDING ON HOSPITAL PROPERTY

Earlier in this chapter, I noted the problems and benefits of renting space in an office building owned by the hospital. A variation of this approach is for a group of doctors to erect their own office building on land leased from the hospital.

Advantages:

1. Overall cost of the project is relatively low, since land is not purchased.

2. Doctors are more independent of hospital control than are those who lease offices in a hospital-owned building.

3. Proximity to hospital reduces doctors' travel time and need to drive in hazardous weather conditions.

4. Access to hospital simplifies special tests and procedures for patients.

5. Equity in building is likely to be salable with little difficulty at doctor's retirement or death.

6. Doctors in other specialties are available for referrals.

7. Hospital's cafeteria and pharmacy are convenient for doctors, staff, and patients.

8. Hospital's switchboard may serve as doctors' answering service.

Disadvantages:

1. Conflict with hospital is possible over duplication of services—lab, X-ray—performed in hospital and in doctors' offices.

2. Design of building may be dictated by hospital.

3. Your investment may be jeopardized if hospital's reputation declines or it moves to a new site.

3
EXPERTS WHO CAN HELP

There are many complex and expensive decisions involved in planning and completing your new office. Mistakes cost money as well as time. You can avoid or minimize them by finding competent people who will act as your advisers. Nine types of advisers are described in this chapter. Depending on the kind of office you are looking for, you may need different combinations of them.

If you want to get the most from your experts, here are a few general rules to follow:

1. Look for the best advisers you can find, not necessarily the cheapest. You'll usually get what you pay for. Always investigate the adviser's track record by speaking to others who have had the same services performed by him.

2. Bring in each consultant right at the *start* of the project. This Is when the most costly and important questions are decided. Be frank when discussing the project with him.

3. Tell the expert *what* you want done, not *how*. Explain your goals, but don't insist on your way of attaining them, at least not until you have heard his solution first. Allow your adviser to come up with his own approach. It may be better than yours.

4. When your consultant does offer satisfactory solutions, insist on their being worked out in painstaking detail. Don't accept only broad concepts. They are generally worthless until the specifics are also presented.

5. At the beginning of your relationship with each consultant, find out exactly how his fee is to be arrived at and when it is to be paid.

6. Try to find experts whose personalities seem to harmonize with yours. You'll have to work closely with these people for many months. Don't saddle yourself with an abrasive person, no matter how talented.

THE ARCHITECT AND/OR THE INTERIOR DESIGNER

Two of the experts most frequently required for the new office are the architect and the interior designer. Though their training is different, their roles can overlap. Occasionally, one or the other performs the functions of both.

An architect's basic function is to design a building, to work out its structural and mechanical needs, and to prepare the necessary plans and specifications for the builder to follow. He also analyzes how the building will be used and plans the arrangement of the walls accordingly. A full discussion of the architect's role is found in Chapter 4.

The interior designer's job usually concerns the design of the indoor space, the creation of an atmosphere or image through the use of furniture, cabinetry, surface finishes (such as floor and wall coverings), fabrics, and accessories. Some interior designers also serve as "interior architects" or space planners for office layouts. A more complete review of the types of interior designers and how to select one can be found in Chapter 38.

If you're erecting a new building you may require the services of both an architect and an interior designer. If so, it's important that they work together from the start of the job in order for you to have a coherent design plan.

EQUIPMENT COMPANIES' OFFICE-PLANNING DEPARTMENTS

Major medical and dental supply firms have office-planning departments that claim to offer some or all of the following services:

☐ advice on location selection;

☐ design of office partitions (space planning);

☐ preparation of drawings for use by builder;

☐ assistance in interior design, furnishing, and decorating;

☐ suggestions for obtaining financing;

☐ advice on equipment selection;

☐ provision of equipment templates and specifications to the builder with electrical and plumbing requirements; and

☐ supervision of contractors and subcontractors.

An evaluation of these services requires an understanding of how these companies operate. They are in business to sell equipment and supplies to doctors. They are eager to establish and to maintain a good-will relationship with you, the doctor-customer. Their office-planning services are a means to this end.

In the past, these services were offered to the doctor without charge in the hope that he would buy equipment from the company. The cost of operating these planning departments has become so expensive, however, that many companies charge for the services unless a large amount of equipment is ordered. A common arrangement now is a flat fee based on the square-foot area of the office or on the number of exam/treatment rooms. If you buy equipment that exceeds a predetermined total price, part or all of the planning fee is waived.

How good are these companies' services? Some of them can be very good if you know what to expect. Some are atrocious. They are best at planning the placement of equipment, in preparing for its installation, and in supervising and doing the actual installation. They also can sometimes refer you to reliable local contractors who have done this type of office construction before. They should know how to guide a builder in such matters as reinforcing walls for the support of wall-hung equipment, how and where to place radiation shielding, and exactly what size wires and pipes are needed for your equipment.

Other aspects of the equipment companies' planning services may not be so successful. In their zeal to satisfy you, they may draw to scale whatever rough sketches you give them of room arrangement, without the critical analysis you'd get from a competent architect. They may pick up glaring errors, but don't expect them to spend days or weeks working out a truly imaginative design for your office layout. They may be interested only in the orthodox arrangement of equipment and may discourage creative planning. Another problem is that some companies push equipment that may not be suitable for the doctor.

The best way to find out about the quality of these services is to get the names of several doctors whose offices were planned by the particular company you're considering. Ask about the competence, reliability, and promptness of the company. If the other doctors were satisfied, you may be, too.

My own feeling is that in some rented suites the supply-house planning department often will be satisfactory, especially if only a few partitions have to be built or moved. However, the cost of establishing a new office is now so high that any project involving substantial interior construction or alteration should have the benefit of an architect or interior architect to help you safeguard your investment. The equipment company can then be called on primarily to supply the detailed information required to prepare the office for equipment installation and, later, to install the equipment.

THE PROFESSIONAL BUSINESS CONSULTANT AND THE REAL-ESTATE CONSULTANT

The professional business consultant (PBC) is a familiar figure in doctors' offices as an adviser on many aspects of practice management and on the doctor's private financial problems. This expert can help you to reach decisions on:

☐ whether you actually need a new office;
☐ what is the best location—with consideration of neighborhood quality and zoning restrictions;
☐ whether to buy, rent, or build;
☐ how to finance the project;
☐ tax considerations;
☐ likely risks and rewards of the whole idea;
☐ how to negotiate for a building site; and
☐ how to negotiate for rental space with a landlord.

While there are other types of advisers who can offer many of the same services, the PBC has the benefit of the experiences of other doctors to draw upon. In addition, he can be completely objective because he has no financial interest in whether you move or whether your building ever goes up.

If you want to erect a building, your PBC's first task will probably be to assemble an analysis of the project, such as the one discussed in Chapter 12. This will include site cost, construction costs, estimated income and expenses of the completed building, possible rental schedules and tax aspects. If this is done with realistic figures, the PBC should be able to tell you whether your idea is worth pursuing.

You can find a business consultant through word-of-mouth referral from other doctors and through the professional business magazines, such as *Medical Economics* or *Dental Management.* These periodicals often publish articles by PBCs. Other sources are the Society of Medical-Dental Management Consultants, 6100 Golden Valley Road, Minneapolis, Minn. 55422, and the Society of Professional Business Consultants, 221 North LaSalle Street, Chicago, Ill. 60601.

When you are trying to decide which of several business consultants to choose, look for one with experience and in-depth knowledge of the type of project you are planning. Always speak to other clients of the adviser to learn about his strong and weak points.

If you're unable or unwilling to engage the services of a PBC, you can sometimes get other help in preparing an investment analysis of a planned building. Accountants and lawyers with extensive real-estate backgrounds can do it, as can certain architects and builders.

If your building project is a very large one, you may benefit by engaging a real-estate consultant or appraiser. This expert, who should *not* be a real-estate broker, will perform the analysis you need and can also be valuable because of his knowledge of real estate in the community. Unfortunately, such people are relatively rare outside the large cities and their suburbs.

The key word is *objectivity.* If your expert has anything to gain by encouraging the project, he's likely to paint too rosy a picture, either consciously or unconsciously. An overoptimistic analysis that highlights the benefits while minimizing the risks is worse than useless. It can lead you to start an enterprise that will leave you with a heavy and long-lasting financial burden.

THE LAWYER

You'll need your attorney's services to advise you on all leases, contracts, mortgages, and partnership agreements before you sign anything; he can suggest the most advantageous form of ownership of the various things you'll need. You must know whether your land, building, equipment, and furnishings should be owned or leased by you as an individual, by you as a member of a partnership, by a trust, by a corporation, or by any of several other possible entities. The attorney should then be able to take the necessary steps to create any such entity and to represent you at local government hearings involving changes of zoning.

You should have a lawyer who has a broad and detailed knowledge of real estate, leases, and tax law. Your new office must be studied in the context of your current needs, your future retirement, and your estate plan.

THE ACCOUNTANT

Your accountant will be needed to help you with:
☐ cash-flow projections;
☐ loan applications;
☐ tax-shelter projections;
☐ tax consequences of proposed actions;
☐ bookkeeping during and after construction; and
☐ monetary details of mortgages, contracts, and other agreements.

THE REAL-ESTATE BROKER

A knowledgeable local realtor is essential when you want to be directed to buildings or condominiums for sale, suitable locations for a proposed building, or available rental space. He must be familiar with neighborhood changes, zoning laws, prevailing rents, land prices, and the availability and cost of mortgage financing.

When in the process of buying land or a building or a condominium, keep in mind that the broker is representing, and is paid by, the seller of the property he shows you. Any comments made by the broker about the suitability of the property for your office should be listened to with the realization that the broker wants to make a sale. Do your own independent investigation of anything he tells you.

When a broker serves as your agent for finding suitable rental space, you may be paying the commission as a percentage of the rent specified in the lease. If you attempt to negotiate a lower rent on the property, the broker may be less than enthusiastic about helping you, for this will serve only to lower his commission.

THE INSURANCE ADVISER

You can choose your regular insurance agent as your adviser. He must know what your risk exposures during construction will be for personal injury and for loss or damage to property. Your adviser should review the insurance coverages of the contractor, the equipment supplier, and, later, the mover. When appropriate, he should recommend supplementary coverages and/or new endorsements on existing policies to protect you throughout construction. The question about who pays when a loss or injury occurs during construction can be difficult to resolve. For example, your builder's insurance may not cover your loss if a fire should destroy some of your equipment in your still incomplete new office. Your insurance agent must help you to fill such gaps.

4

YOU NEED
AN ARCHITECT

Once you've made the decision to build, lease, or renovate an office the most immediate question is: Do I need an architect?

You've heard the usual stories: One doctor had a builder who was "just as good" as an architect; another borrowed a friend's plans because "architects are too expensive"; you "don't really need one"; and "they all want to build a Taj Mahal."

My answer, based on firsthand experience in rented, renovated, and newly constructed offices, is a definite Yes. You do need an architect.

A properly chosen architect can make the entire new-office project a tolerable or even a pleasant one instead of an ulcer-producing nightmare that leaves you swearing, "Never again!"

The functions that most people identify with the architect are the design of the building and the floor plan of the office. While these are certainly important, there are others that I've found at least as valuable:

1. A good architect provides fully detailed architectural and mechanical working drawings and specifications. They are needed by the bank for deciding on financing and by the builder for submitting a bid. The more complete this material is, the fewer misunderstandings there will be during construction.

2. The architect can find the right builders to bid on the project, firms with which he has worked in the past. This is one of the most critical parts of an architect's services. A builder who obtains the contract for your job through an architect will be eager to please that architect, for the latter can be an important source of future jobs to him.

3. The competent architect reviews the bids and negotiates contract details with the bidders. This is the stage at which he can earn a large part of his fee.

Skillful revision of floor plans, changes of materials, or other relatively small adjustments can produce savings worth thousands of dollars. Your architect should make recommendations regarding which bid should be accepted and offer guidance on the terms of the contract with the builder.

4. The architect is the one who can resolve the inevitable disagreements between yourself and the builder. In effect, he is your interpreter; his presence in this role can avoid long and unpleasant arguments with the builder. In our own project, which involved both renovation and new construction and which lasted more than six months, we never exchanged harsh words with the builder. When any disagreement arose we each, separately, spoke to the architect and generally abided by his suggestion. Remember that the architect must be fair to the builder, too. It is considered unethical for an architect to favor one side over the other.

Suppose you decide not to engage an architect and you are dealing directly with a builder. A disagreement arises; you and the builder differ in your interpretation of the plans. Tempers flare. The dispute escalates. You threaten to stop payment until changes are made. The builder responds by threatening to walk off the job until he is paid for the changes.

Such disagreements with the builder are likely to be "no-win" situations. They yield only indigestion, sleepless nights, and long-lasting hard feelings. I learned this from people who have been there.

A good architect speaks the builder's language and knows your job intimately. Let him win your points for you or else explain to you why what you are asking the builder to do is unreasonable.

5. There are other services that your architect can provide. He should:

☐ be available for all necessary meetings with you, and should not be subject to temperamental outbursts at these meetings if you do not accept some of his suggestions;

☐ promptly send you copies of all drawings produced or altered as a result of each meeting;

☐ assemble, and submit for your approval, samples of all materials being considered for use;

☐ retain consultants as needed;

□ aid in preparation of the contract;

□ be familiar with all local building codes and zoning restrictions and be sure that your building and office will not violate any of them;

□ inspect the construction at regular intervals (which should be specified in his contract) and be available for phone consultation as needed; and

□ approve payments when justified and delay approval of payments until he is satisfied that the work has been done properly.

Note that the architect's role is to *inspect*, not *supervise*.

Supervision is the day-to-day job of the contractor or his foreman. The architect, on the other hand, should observe or inspect the work periodically to be sure that your interests are protected. The frequency of his visits need not be based on a specified number of days. Instead, it can be keyed to the progress of the work. If you are erecting a building, for example, he should visit the site when the excavation is complete, when the foundation is finished, and at various stages thereafter. If the construction is in an existing building, he should inspect as soon as the framing is completed, when all rough-ins are done, when the wallboard is up, and later at intervals during the finishing process.

SELECTING AN ARCHITECT

If you're now convinced that you should engage an architect for your project, where do you find one? What criteria should you use in selecting him? What is a fair fee for his services?

Before I offer specific suggestions, a general comment is appropriate. Your new-office project is going to be time-consuming and expensive. It can also be very unpleasant if you select the wrong people to work with. Don't minimize the effort needed to find the right architect. Ample time spent at this stage in searching out the best available person will save many hours and possibly thousands of dollars later.

Direct referral is the most frequently used method of finding an architect. Every health professional in your area who has recently moved into a newly built or renovated office should be asked about his architect. I suggest inquiring primarily among health professionals—dentists, physicians, podiatrists—since you want an architect familiar with this kind of construction, its design, and its mechanical needs.

Drive around the community looking for medical and/or dental buildings. Don't seek only new structures. Look also for renovated older buildings. Look at friends' offices in rented suites that were designed by an architect.

Criteria for selecting an architect

As you consider each prospect, keep in mind that the ideal architect combines the originality, sensitivity, and talent of an artist with the practical attitudes of the cost-conscious businessman. Moreover, he is someone whose temperament is compatible with yours; not just at your first interview when he may be trying to impress you, but later during the stressful periods of planning and construction. Of course, you can't expect to find the perfect architect, but the following guidelines can help you find the best available to you. For each architect you interview:

1. Visit his office and ask to see models or photographs of jobs similar to yours. Note the addresses and visit those buildings later.

2. As you talk to him, ask yourself if you'll be able to communicate with this person for many hours at a time, relying on his judgment in matters that involve the investment of many thousands of dollars. Here is where your skill in evaluating people will be tested.

3. Ask about his fees. Is he forthright in telling you how much he will charge, and what his fee does and does not include? Or does he mumble, "Don't worry; we'll work it out later," or words to that effect? (Warning: That expression, "Don't worry . . .," coming from anyone involved in your new-office project, should immediately alert you to the possibility of impending disaster. Freely translated, the phrase means, "Get off my back, Doc. I haven't figured that out yet.") We'll have more to say about architects' fees later.

4. Go to see his work even if it means travel and expense. Try to arrange a meeting with the owners at the same time. What was their experience with him? Was he easy to work with? Did he meet deadlines? Was he conscious of the need to keep costs down? Were his estimates realistic about the time and cost of construction? Was he helpful in selecting a builder and in negotiating the builder's contract? Did he visit the construction site to the extent called for in his contract? Did they have any problems with him? Did he work well with the equipment supplier? Would they engage him again for another job?

If the office you are visiting is in a new building, it is useful—but often difficult—to find out if the *actual construction cost* of the building was close to the *appraised market value.* The latter figure was assigned to the building by the bank's appraiser when the construction loan was negotiated. This comparison suggests whether the architect was able to design a structure that could be built at a reasonable cost. If the two figures are far apart it could mean that the architect included special features that added substantially to the cost without adding to the building's value. This in turn can result in an insufficient construction loan, requiring the owners to put up much more cash than anticipated. Many owners may be unwilling to discuss these financial details with you, especially if you're a stranger to them, but you may be able to pick up hints of dissatisfaction from the way they speak.

Your choice of an architect should not be based entirely on his past performance in designing professional offices or buildings. Sometimes an experienced architect can be inflexible; a younger, more enthusiastic person may be motivated to research your project thoroughly and to come up with imaginative solutions.

In the final analysis, you'll probably choose your architect because you trust him, because you have confidence in his judgment, and because your ability to communicate with each other tells you that this is the right person.

The architect's fee

When you need an architect for interior design or consultation services—not a building—his fee may be calculated on an hourly basis within a range of $50 to $125 an hour. Another method of determining the fee is "time against an upset"—an hourly rate with a maximum fee specified. A third type of fee arrangement is on a square-foot basis. This is the way some space planners and interior architects charge for their services.

Your consultant could use any one of these methods or a combination of them. A fourth approach is a percentage of cabinetwork cost. If the architect must draw many complicated detail drawings for a casework wall, his fee could be a percentage of its cost, plus perhaps a flat additional amount.

Since so many variations in fee structure are possible, you'd better find out early how your expert will want to be paid.

The usual range of architects' fees for designing a building is 7 to 12 percent of the "budgeted construction cost" (not including cost of the land), including engineering fees and periodic inspections of the work. The higher the budget, the lower will be the architect's percentage. Thus the fee could be 10 to 12 percent for a $150,000 building and 9 percent for a $500,000 building.

Notice that I used the expression "budgeted construction cost" (or budget) rather than actual construction cost. Early in the planning for your office you'll have to decide, with the architect, what you want and how much you are willing to pay. Once he agrees to design your building and to "bring it in" (get it built) for that amount, you have arrived at a budget. With one exception, the architect's percentage should be based on the budgeted cost only, not on the actual cost of construction.

Here's why: If poor judgment on the part of the architect brings the cost of your building 50 percent above the budgeted cost, he should not benefit by getting a percentage of the overrun. Although some increase in costs beyond what was expected seems to creep into virtually every job, a good architect should be able to keep this increase down to no more than 10 or 15 percent.

On the other hand—and this is the one exception—if *you* insist on substantial changes in the plans after construction has started, then the architect is justified in demanding an extra fee for revising the plans. However, if all of the bids are considerably higher than the agreed-upon budget, the architect should be willing to redesign the building to bring down its cost.

If, by some miracle, the architect brings in the building you want *below* the budgeted cost estimate, then he should still get the agreed-upon percentage of the budget. He's earned it.

I'd be wary of an architect whose fee scale is very much below that of other architects in the area. This could mean that he's using stock plans, that he will do few inspections, or that he will cut corners in other ways.

The manner of payment of the architect's fee may seem unusual to you. He'll probably ask for approximately 80 percent of his fee divided over a number of weeks or months during the planning stage, before any construction is done. The last 20 percent is paid during construction for his inspection of the work. This arrangement is fair, because the major part of his work ends when working drawings and specifications are finished and a contractor's bid is accepted.

The architect's contract

If your architect is a member of the American Institute of Architects he'll probably prepare an A.I.A. contract for your signature. This should spell out what he will do, how his fee is to be established, when it is to be paid, how frequently he is to visit the site, and other details.

Although it's advisable to have your attorney review the document, the specific language of the contract is far less important than the choice of the person. In other words, if you've found the right architect, just a handshake is enough. The purpose of a written contract is to avoid later misunderstandings by listing the obligations of each party. Remember, too, that the preprinted contract is negotiable. Sections can be changed, if necessary, for added clarity.

There are three other fees that relate to the architect's work, but are often billed separately:

Reproductions. You will have to pay the cost of copies of all plans, drawings, and specifications submitted to you or to the builders on your behalf. This figure can easily run to more than $500 on even a small office building.

Engineering. For a medium- or large-size new building, your architect should retain a structural and a mechanical engineer for planning steel work, heating, air conditioning, and electrical needs. The bill for engineering consultations can range from hundreds to thousands of dollars. Sometimes it is included in the architect's fee, sometimes not. Find out. If it isn't included, try to get an estimate of engineering costs from the architect early in the planning process. If you are going to renovate an old building, the engineer may be needed to evaluate the existing mechanical systems in the building.

Surveys. If you're erecting a new building, you probably paid for a survey at the time you bought the land. But the architect will ask you for a topographic survey (or *topo*) as well. This shows the contours of the land, trees, and other surface and subsurface features that he will have to consider.

II
THE ALTERNA-TIVES TO BUILDING: FIRST GUIDELINES

5
IF YOU LEASE

This chapter offers hints to guide you in what to do and what to avoid in leasing a new office. Following chapters in Section II provide guidelines for other routes to new quarters. Construction of a new building is more complicated. It's treated separately in Section III.

Consider each of the alternatives as thoroughly and as unemotionally as you can. Look into *all* details and get expert help before you sign anything.

If you're serious about leasing space, first consider the building. Is it well located for easy patient access? If it's in a suburban area, is the parking adequate even at the busiest times of the day? Does the building's appearance appeal to you? Does it look well built, clean, and well maintained? Are the service people, such as elevator operators and porters, courteous and neatly dressed?

Before you negotiate your lease, talk to other tenants in the building, especially other doctors. What has been their experience with the landlord? Is he a reasonable person to deal with? Does he fulfill his commitments? Does the building maintenance staff keep it in good repair? Do the heating, air conditioning, and plumbing systems work well? Did they have any problems in obtaining the necessary electric and plumbing connections when their offices were built? Are the halls, elevators, windows, and washrooms kept clean? Do the washrooms always have adequate soap and paper goods? Have there been any problems with burglary or other crime in the building?

Talk to the landlord or his renting agent. The welcome you receive will depend largely on the state of the office rental market at the time. If the building is almost full and there is little other rental space available in the area, you can expect a cool reception. The landlord will not be disposed to grant many concessions in order to get you as a tenant. But if his building has a substantial amount of unoccupied space, your bargaining position becomes much stronger. Before you negotiate with him, try to find out from other tenants if there are many offices vacant and for how long.

Landlords have considerably more experience in negotiating with tenants than you have in dealing with landlords. When you bring up some matter discussed below, the landlord may try to put you down for doing so, as if you are overstepping an inviolable boundary. Ignore that response. It's a tactic used by many negotiators. Your success in getting what you want will be determined by the strength of your bargaining position and by your skill as a "horse trader." (For a thorough discussion of negotiating strategies and tactics, see *The Art of Negotiating* by Gerard I. Nierenberg, New York: Hawthorn, 1968.)

The questions that follow are appropriate for many different kinds of rental situations. You'll have to choose the ones that are right for you. Most of the points mentioned are summarized in the worksheet at the end of this chapter.

I'm not a lawyer. Any agreements with the landlord about these points should be carefully worded in close collaboration with your own attorney.

1. What is the rent per square foot per year? Caution: Ask *how* the square footage is calculated. The square-foot total you're interested in is the *usable* footage. The landlord thinks in terms of *rentable* footage, which may be quite different. Some include the thickness of the outside walls of the building in your square-foot total. Others say you have to pay for footage outside your own office. They charge for your share of common areas on the floor.

Example: A commercial office building floor has a total of 5,000 square feet. Washrooms, hallways, and utility closet occupy 800 square feet. There remains 4,200 square feet of usable space. The ratio of rentable to usable space on this floor will be 5,000 to 4,200, or a "load factor" of about 1.2. To obtain 1,000 square feet of usable space in this building you must multiply your desired usable footage by 1.2. Thus you have to pay rent on 1,200 square feet even though you use only 1,000 in your office. This practice may vary from one community to another and even from one building to another in the same city. Measure the usable footage *yourself* in the building or on architectural prints. Two doctors in partnership were told that their suite in a large midtown Manhattan building contained 1,700 usable square feet. Their measurements showed that they were getting only 1,450 square feet. Don't rely on plans that are not drawn to scale. Some renting agents use undimensioned drawings in their negotiations with prospective tenants.

2. Does the local zoning code permit the practice of your profession in the building? In some towns, the codes strictly limit where professionals may practice. If there are no other doctors in the building, find out if the building's certificate of occupancy permits you to practice there. Some health departments limit the number of people who may be in a reception room at one time. Does the local building department place any restrictions on floor load capacity? This could limit your use of heavy equipment.

3. Will you be responsible for maintenance or repairs in any part of the building other than in your office, such as the central heating or air-conditioning equipment? Any repairs that will be your responsibility should be spelled out in detail. All others should be at the landlord's expense.

4. Will your obligation to pay rent stop if the premises become unfit for use, such as after a fire or as a result of storm damage, or if the building is condemned by the local municipality? It should.

5. Are there any "escalators" tied to the rent, such as increases in rent when there are increases in the building's operating costs, increases in the Consumer Price Index, increases in real-estate taxes, or even increases in your office income? All of these have been tried by landlords in different areas. Avoid them if possible, but recognize that in these inflationary times landlords may insist on such a clause. Usually these escalators run only one way: up! In other words, your rent won't go below the minimum level at which it began, but it can go higher, depending on what activates the escalator.

If an escalator clause is unavoidable, learn exactly how it operates or you could be in for some unpleasant surprises. If it's based on a pass-through of operating costs, find out how these are calculated and whether you'll have to take the landlord's word for the amount of the increase. There are some tricky ploys used by landlords, such as using a time before the building was fully rented as the base period for calculating future increases in operating expenses. Also, landlords know that an audit of their books will be very expensive for the tenant. That's why they may say glibly that you can feel free to corroborate their statements of cost increases.

Remember, this is a negotiable item. It's an area in which you should exercise your bargaining skill as well as you can.

6. Who is responsible for insurance on the property? You should carry the insurance within your own office, but the landlord should carry the insurance on the public areas, such as hallway, lobbies, and elevators.

7. Is there any limitation on the amount of electricity you can draw from existing power lines? Some areas have limited electrical power, and this could affect your practice.

8. Is there a grace period for the payment of rent (such as 5 days), or will you be in default if you do not pay by the first of each month?

9. If the building is under construction, is there a specified completion date? Your rent in a new building should not begin until you are able to use your office. Other important parts of the building, such as elevators, parking lots, and washrooms, should be usable as well.

10. What services will be provided and how frequently? Ask about office cleaning, window washing, floor waxing, garbage removal, exterminator services, snow plowing, lawn maintenance, and painting.

11. Will you have the use of storage areas in the building outside your own office? How much space? How far from your office? Are they always accessible? Without any additional rent?

12. What security systems are provided? Who, besides yourself and your staff, will have a key to your office?

13. What utilities are provided and which will be your responsibility? There should be a separate meter for every utility you will have to pay for.

14. What interior temperatures are maintained at various seasons of the year? Is the heat and/or the air conditioning turned off at night? At what time? Commercial office buildings must comply with maximum and minimum temperatures for energy conservation. Health-care offices are exempt from this, but you may have to supply supplemental heating and/or cooling yourself.

15. Will you have access to your suite at whatever hours you choose?

16. How many parking spaces will be guaranteed for use by you and your patients? If the building isn't fully rented, what looks like ample parking space now could turn out to be entirely inadequate when all the offices are occupied. You'll need space for each doctor, each staff member, and for as many patients as you have in the office at peak hours.

17. Will you have the right to sublet your suite to other practitioners? Will the landlord have to approve? Try to avoid this, or at least have the lease specify that the landlord won't be unreasonable in withholding consent.

18. If the lease is to contain renewal options, be sure you clearly understand how many months before renewal you have to notify the landlord in writing of your intention not to renew. You could be obligated to pay five or more years of rent because you didn't let him know in time.

19. Will there be any limitation to the placement of your name on the building's directory or on your office door? Some leases prohibit signs of any kind. Can a doctor who subleases your office list his name on the directory?

There are two basic modes of office rental, sometimes known as *finished* and *shell*. A *shell* is an office in which just the four outer walls of the suite plus air conditioning, elevators, and basic utilities are provided. The tenant arranges and pays directly for all construction and decorating.

In a *finished* office, the landlord takes responsibility for basic construction and decoration, based on plans provided by the tenant. The tenant pays for this through an increase in the annual rent per square foot.

While it might appear to your advantage to have the landlord pay for necessary construction, this may not be true. The resulting increase in the annual rent creates a high *base rent*, to which most escalator clauses are tied. When increases are demanded at lease-renewal time, they'll be calculated as a percentage of the base rent. Thus, it may be better for you to keep the base rent low, borrow the needed money, and pay for the alterations yourself. One instance in which it's better to have the landlord do the work occurs when your own lines of credit are severely stretched by other borrowing and you'd have trouble getting funds for construction.

In your discussion with the landlord, find out if you have such a choice. Here are some of the issues you can negotiate:

If you do the alteration (you rent a shell):

1. Will you be responsible for restoring the premises to their original state when you move out? When you leave, will you be able to take with you any of the built-ins you install?

2. Can you use contractors and workmen of your own choosing? Some landlords insist on your selecting a builder from a limited list of names.

3. Will your workmen be able to work in the building whenever they choose? If they are nonunion, will they be harassed by union workers in the building? (For guidelines on negotiating a contract with the builder, see Chapter 35.)

If the landlord does the alteration (the office is "finished"):

1. What exactly is the work to be done by the landlord? This should be contained in a separate part of your lease, called a *work letter.* It should state in detail the items and the work the landlord will do. The more complete this description, the fewer will be the problems that arise later. The work letter should be accompanied by the necessary specifications and plans drawn to scale by your architect or office designer. These should be as detailed as possible and include all partitions, doors, flooring, ceiling, lighting, wall covering, electrical, and plumbing needs. (All of these are discussed in separate chapters.) If you simply hand the landlord or his builder a rough sketch and say, "This is what I want," you're asking for trouble. And the trouble won't become apparent until it's very costly to change.

2. Who will provide the insurance during this construction?

3. What grade of materials will be used? Building materials come in several grades. In large commercial office buildings, one particular grade (often called the *building standard)* is used for each item. If you want a better grade you'll have to pay extra for it. For example, if the light switches normally used are the standard up-and-down toggle switches, but you want decorative push button switches, there will be an extra charge for each one. Find out in advance what is the usual grade of each item and what each change will cost.

4. If the landlord provides carpeting, how frequently will it be replaced? Is the quality specified?

5. Will you have to start paying rent if the alterations are not completed on time? You shouldn't.

6. Who will guarantee the finished work, the landlord or his contractor, and for how long?

7. Will you be able to make alterations later as your needs change?

TABLE 5-1

Office Space Evaluation Worksheet

Address: _____

Owner
(or agent): _____ Phone: _____

Type of building:
  Medical building/commercial building/
    single office/house

Building setting:
  Urban/surburban/medical center
    area/professional park

Location:
Convenience to current patients: _____

Potential for new patients: _____

Convenience to hospitals: _____

Staff privileges at hospitals: _____

Public transportation
  serving area: _____

Access to thoroughfares: _____

Office facilities:

Zoning OK? _____

Parking: On premises/adjacent/on street/metered

Adequacy of parking: _____

Size of suite: _____ sq. ft.

Extra rent for public areas? _____

Room for expansion? _____

Partitioning needed: _____ linear feet

Partitioning, other construction
  to be paid for by: _____

Utilities and services offered:

Heat: _____ No. of zones: _____

  Temps maintained: Day _____ Night _____

Air conditioning: _____ No. of zones: _____

  Temps maintained: Day _____ Night _____

continued

Electric wiring capacity: _____

Elevator: _____

Access to building limited at night? _____

Office cleaning: _____ Frequency: _____

Window washing: _____ Frequency: _____

Floor waxing: _____ Frequency: _____

Garbage removal: _____ Frequency: _____

Security systems: _____

Extra storage available:

   Terms of use: _____

Lease terms:

Annual rent: $ _____ per sq. ft. per year on _____ sq. ft.

Monthly rent: _____ Grace period? _____

Escalator clause? _____

   Based on: _____

Length of lease: _____

Option to renew? _____

When must landlord be notified? _____

Option to sublet? _____

Escape clause? _____ Penalty: _____

Decorating: What? _____ Frequency: _____

Restore to original when moving out? _____

Who carries insurance? _____

Does rent continue if premises are unfit for use? ____

Who pays for repairs in office? _____

   In common areas of building? _____

If building is under construction,
   when does rent start? _____

Signs: Outside: _____

      Building directory: _____

      Office door: _____

The landlord will probably hand you what he refers to as "our standard office lease." Beware! This preprinted document is written solely for the benefit of landlords. Read it carefully, review it with your lawyer, and have it changed to conform to the agreement you negotiated with the landlord. If you are in a good bargaining position, every part of a lease is negotiable.

In addition to the points mentioned earlier in this chapter, your lawyer will probably want the lease to describe clearly the space to be rented, the amount of rent and how it is to be paid, the length of the lease, any agreed-on escalator clauses and/or options, your right to assign the office, and the conditions for terminating the lease (such as your death or disability).

There are some tax considerations related to capital expenses (such as construction, equipment, and furniture) and the length of your lease. These should be reviewed by a competent accountant before you sign the document.

Finally, two more comments about renting: If any borrowed property belonging to the landlord, such as furniture, is to remain in your office, have it described in detail in the lease and take photos of it to show its condition when you start to use it.

Try to obtain more office space than you think you need, or at least get the "right of first refusal" on any adjacent space that may become available.

Make extra copies of Table 5-1 and use them to compare the features of the buildings you visit.

6
IF YOU SUBLEASE

Be wary of the doctor who is subletting the space if he says, "We don't need a written agreement. We can work the details out later." His understanding of those details will almost certainly differ from yours. Write down everything that's agreed upon. You may feel that you do not need the formality of a written sublease, but it's prudent to prepare a letter or memorandum of understanding of your rights and obligations.

Be sure your *written* agreement with the subletting doctor covers at least these points:

1. Does it assure that he has the landlord's permission to sublet to you.

2. Does it list the number of hours per day and days per week you may use the office. Will the building be open if you wish to work during early morning or late evening hours? Which days of the week will it be available?

3. Does it provide for secretarial and assistant services? If you will depend on the other doctor's office help to assist you, find out if there's any conflict on holidays. Will they expect to be off when you might wish to work?

4. Will you use the other doctor's phone and answering service or will you provide your own?

5. For how long a period will the specified rent remain the same?

6. Who provides disposable and expendable items, such as paper towels or cups, head-rest or table covers, pencils, paper clips, and other supplies?

7. How much advance notice must be given by either party to terminate the agreement?

8. Find out what your insurance needs are. Some malpractice insurers, for example, insist that all doctors working in the same office have coverage by the same company, even though the doctors have separate practices.

7
IF YOU BUY A CONDOMINIUM

Review the section in Chapter 5 about renting and lease negotiation, because many of the points made there are pertinent to the condominium situation, especially those relating to building operation and maintenance. As a part owner of the building, you have different responsibilities than if you were a tenant, but all of these should be clearly spelled out in the purchase documents. Check the worksheet at the end of Chapter 5 for appropriate items.

In addition, you should get satisfactory answers on these points:

1. What are the taxes? Can you verify them independently? If the building is not yet up, how realistic is the organizer's estimate? Developers of real-estate projects tend to be overoptimistic in projecting future expenses for prospective owners. Can you discover the taxes on similar units at the assessor's office?

2. What will be the monthly operating and maintenance costs? How will they be apportioned among the unit owners of the building? On a square-foot basis? What happens if one or more occupants default on these payments? Is there an escrow account to limit this problem?

3. What mortgage terms are available?

4. Will you have any control over the purchasers of other units in the building? Is there a limit on the number of practices in any one specialty? Will you be restricted as to type of buyer for your unit when you want to sell?

5. Do you have an attorney who is well informed about condos? In many states, the paperwork is complex and time-consuming.

6. If the condo office is in an existing building, was an appraisal done?

7. Do you know your insurance responsibilities? Some condominium associations have quirks in their insurance coverage over what is provided by the owner of an individual unit and what the association provides.

8. Does a condominium office make sense as an investment?

8
IF YOU RENOVATE AN OLD BUILDING

Look for a building that is in a stable neighborhood, preferably within a few blocks of the hospital; this will make your building easier to sell when that time comes.

Get your architect *before* you buy the building. There are so many problems in old structures that you'll need the architect's expertise right from the start.

Carefully investigate the local zoning and building codes. The local building department or building inspector should be able to answer these questions:

1. Is the building in a zone that permits professional offices? Many older homes, which might be suitable for conversion into offices, are in zones for residential use only. A doctor may practice in a residential zone only if he also lives in the same building.

2. Is the community preparing a master plan that may change the uses permitted on the property you're interested in?

3. If professional offices are prohibited in the neighborhood, how liberal is the local zoning board in granting variances or changes of zoning? My partner and I had very little trouble in obtaining a variance to convert an old house into an office. Yet, in some communities, such changes are virtually unobtainable. Opposition from nearby residents often persuades the board to refuse a change of zone. (Zoning is discussed in greater detail in Chapter 15.)

4. What about parking? Is there a zoning requirement for a specific number of on-site parking spaces? If so, is there room on the property for that many spaces? A good rule of thumb is to try to have eight to 10 spaces *per doctor* for the cars of the doctor, staff, and patients in a busy practice. Is on-street parking permitted? Don't rely on it. It can change at the whim of local officials.

5. Does the local building or health code have any restrictions that might present problems? You'd be unpleasantly surprised if you were told that the health code strictly limited the number of people who could occupy your waiting room at any one time. Are there any special limitations on the use of X-ray machines, on the installation of nitrous oxide analgesia equipment, or on the amount of electricity you use? Is the house connected to a sewer line or to a septic tank? If there is a septic tank, will a sewer hookup be required?

6. Has the building you're interested in been cited by the building department for any violations of local codes or statutes? Have they been corrected? (Such violations may also be uncovered during a title search.)

7. Is there a certificate of occupancy on record? This is an official statement from the local building inspector that the structure met local building requirements at some time in the past and could be occupied. If the building is very old, however, there may not be a certificate in the records.

8. Do the zoning codes permit converting part of the building into apartments if the building is large enough? Residential tenants can be sources of income. Their presence adds to the security of the building.

Order an inspection and obtain a detailed report on the building by your architect and/or an engineer. The report should include:

☐ structural soundness of walls, floors, and roof;
☐ condition of mechanical systems: plumbing, heating, electrical (sometimes it will be cheaper to replace existing systems rather than repair them);
☐ evidence of termites;
☐ type of wall construction (how difficult will it be to move partitions?);
☐ insulation;
☐ moisture problems;
☐ soil conditions (if new construction will be needed).

Discuss with your architect how much construction is needed to provide a desirable floor plan. In some cases, so many changes are necessary that it's less expensive to demolish the structure to its foundation and then build, assuming that the location is a good one. In other situations, it may be worthwhile to have a demolition contractor come in and remove those parts of the building's interior that must be changed *before* you put the final plans and specifications out for bids. The advantage is that prospective bidders will have fewer surprises awaiting them inside the old walls, and their bids may be lower.

If you are thinking of renovating a building with a view toward renting space to other doctors, be aware that you'd risk the same kind of calamity that befell Dr. John P. Callan, a Hartford, Conn., psychiatrist. In his article, "Well, my office building *seemed* like a great investment," in *Medical Economics*, January 21, 1980, Dr. Callan described what happened after he purchased a three-story, 60-year-old building near the local hospital. He moved in and hoped to rent three vacant offices to other doctors.

"The hospital suddenly entered the real-estate market," Dr. Callan wrote, "purchasing a neighboring insurance company building and several doctors' buildings. Ironically, I learned of this when invited to contribute to a nonprofit corporation established to take over the buildings.

"The local physician rental market folded. I was only one of several doctors stuck with unrentable property. One doctor-owner lamented, 'I saw my retirement annuity vanish.'"

Speak to the neighbors. A few phone calls or personal visits can tell you quickly whether there is likely to be opposition to your obtaining a zoning change. In addition, long-time neighbors can often tell you the history of the structure. You may not get interesting bits of information in any other way.

Check with the local utility companies about whether they've had many calls to this building in the recent past. Have there been gas leaks or underground water leaks?

Your attorney should check the deed to the property. Are there any covenants or easements (discussed in Chapter 15) that may limit your use of the building or the land?

Ask your accountant if the rehabilitation of the old building would make you eligible for tax credits under the Revenue Act of 1978.

If you do find an old building that seems suitable for renovation, read Chapter 62. It's a brief account of our experience with converting a 125-year-old structure for use as an office.

9
IF YOU ENLARGE YOUR EXISTING OFFICE

Be sure your landlord won't place obstacles in your way. Much higher rent or new lease restrictions could make expansion considerably less attractive.

Find an architect or interior architect who has experience in this line. You are living dangerously if you engage a builder directly, without other advice. Your expert should inspect the building to determine if the changes you seek are feasible or if alternatives are available.

He should do a review of existing wall, floor, and ceiling construction and a study of the location of utilities. For example, high-rise office buildings have *wet stacks*—vertical columns containing plumbing lines. All plumbing installations must be connected to these stacks. The horizontal piping for each floor usually runs in the space between the floor and the dropped ceiling of the floor below. A "simple" shift of your equipment to a new location may not be simple at all in relation to the existing plumbing.

Check the building-code requirements. Your renovation has to comply with these regulations. If you ignore them, you take the chance that a building inspector will refuse to let you use the premises until corrections are made.

Perhaps most important, you'll have to plan the construction in such a way as to minimize disruption of your practice. There are several ways to do this.

1. Sometimes, virtually all work is completed in the new space while the existing office continues to function. When the new area is completed, the entire practice moves in, while the workmen move to the old section. Finally, the two sections are joined by breaking through the intervening wall. This approach has the advantage of reducing problems of noise and dirt pollution at first. It's unlikely that the new section will serve all your needs while construction goes on in the old office. Also, the connection between the two will probably have to be made sooner than you'd like. This means that you'll have to put up with noise, dust, odors, and utility cutoffs for days or weeks as the work goes on.

2. You may decide to close your office completely for whatever time is needed to do the work. This way, you escape the nuisance of disruptions while you're in the office, and it may be the best way to solve the problem if the alterations won't take much time. If you can use another doctor's office temporarily, fine. But there are two dangers in this approach:

First, don't go off on vacation while the work is being done unless you have an exceptionally knowledgeable and competent staff; someone must be there to answer the questions that inevitably arise. Murphy's Law—"anything that can go wrong, will go wrong"—has its corollaries in the construction industry. Constant vigilance is the only prevention and cure.

Second, don't take seriously the builder's estimate of the time he'll take to complete the work. Builders are notoriously overoptimistic when discussing a proposed job. Strikes, shortages of materials, and the unavailability of skilled labor all cause long, unforeseen delays. Also, the builder and you may not be thinking in the same terms. He says he needs two weeks. To you, this means that in two weeks you can have your wallpaper hung, carpeting laid, and equipment installed. To him, it means that he can finish the demolition and most of the heavy construction work in that time. Very few doctors I've spoken to have had builders whose time projections were realistic. My own experience is that these estimates should be multiplied by a "delay factor" of two or three.

3. Another possibility is to have all the work done at night and on weekends. With this method, however, you can expect excessive labor costs.

Be sure you work out the details and likely costs with your architect before you approach the landlord. You'll have to figure out how high a rent increase you can absorb without the total expense becoming prohibitive. You may find that moving to a new location is a better option, after all.

10
IF YOU BUY A HOME-OFFICE COMBINATION

Be sure you've looked squarely at all the disadvantages of the home-office combination as outlined in Chapter 2. Don't proceed unless you're willing to accept them.

1. Check the zoning in the area. Will it permit another doctor to practice with you—or instead of you—if he doesn't live there?

2. Is the property large enough to expand the building if you need more office space later? The size of the lot in square feet is only part of what you need to know. Equally important is the building setback requirement in the area. This is the minimum number of feet that any part of a building must, according to the local zoning laws, be from the nearest boundary of the property. There's more on such requirements in Chapter 15.

Get expert help for the renovation of the part of the building that is to be your office. Unless you're buying a place with a functioning office that has a suitable layout, you'd better get an experienced architect. Then follow the procedures outlined in this book for creating any office.

11
FINANCING YOUR CONSTRUCTION, EQUIPMENT, AND FURNITURE

If you've now decided where and how to set up your office, you'd better start thinking about how to pay for it. All of the choices discussed in the preceding chapters, except subleasing an equipped office, require a substantial outlay for equipment, furniture, and decorating. If construction is also needed, you'll have to add that cost as well. As one who has recently been through it, I can tell you that the dollar amounts soon reach breathtaking proportions.

"Buy everything for cash only!"

"Leasing makes the most sense!"

"Take a bank loan for as long as you can!"

The professional business magazines frequently carry articles and advertisements extolling one approach or another to financing construction, equipment, and furniture. Since it's important to make a rational decision, let's look at some of the possible options:

Cash purchase with your own capital. If you, your partnership, or your professional corporation has a large amount of accumulated cash, you might use this money to buy your new equipment. You'll get the benefit of the investment tax credit, and each year you'll get a depreciation deduction. If you have the cash, this is usually the least expensive option in the total number of dollars paid out, and possibly in the net cost over a 10-year period also, despite the loss of interest on the cash invested.

A variation of this approach is, in effect, to borrow the money from yourself by using separate entities as borrower and lender. Your accountant and attorney may be able to set this up so that as borrower you pay tax-deductible interest, while for you as lender, the interest income is tax-deferred.

Cash purchase with borrowed money. This approach puts inflation to work for you in two ways: You are converting cash with shrinking purchasing power into tangibles, and you are using someone else's cash. As the dollar's value drops, each succeeding repayment of your loan is made with less valuable dollars than the previous one. If the interest rate you pay is the same or less than the inflation rate, your loan is, in effect, costing you nothing. Meanwhile, your own cash can be earning income elsewhere.

Since you are making an outright purchase, the tax situation with respect to depreciation and the investment-tax credit is probably the same as in our first option. In addition, the interest on your loan is deductible. The total cash outlay here is probably higher than it is when you purchase with your own cash—because you must pay interest on the loan—but less than it is in a lease.

Leasing. A leasing company buys the equipment you select and then leases it to you for a specified length of time. The total dollar amount that you pay over the term of the lease is greater than in either of our first two options, for the leasing company must add its overhead and profit to the cost of the equipment plus financing charges. This is partly compensated for by the fact that the entire lease payment is tax-deductible. You can write off greater amounts each year than if you purchase the equipment.

At the end of the lease term, however, the equipment still belongs to the leasing company. You can probably buy it then at a reduced price, but be careful. Unless this part of the lease is carefully drawn, the I.R.S. may take the position that the whole deal was just an installment purchase and then disallow some of the tax deductions.

Two other alternatives at the end of the lease are a new lease at a lower monthly rate, assuming that the equipment is still usable, or replacement with new equipment and a new lease.

One aspect of leasing often emphasized by the leasing companies is that since a lease is technically not a loan, it won't impair your credit lines for other borrowing. But, like a loan, a lease is an obligation to pay a fixed dollar amount per month for a given number of months. If you apply for a substantial loan for some other purpose, your banker will carefully investigate your financial position and cash flow. He may consider your equipment lease as just one more drain on your ability to repay the new loan.

Seriously consider leasing equipment if:

1. You don't have large reserves of cash, and your credit lines are already fully extended for other reasons. Be sure, however, that your cash flow will allow you to cover the lease payments in addition to your other obligations. If you're already loaded with debt, many leasing companies will have nothing to do with you.

2. The necessary money simply isn't available from conventional lenders because of a credit crunch. Large leasing companies can often obtain funds in the money markets at times when you, as an individual, cannot.

3. You have the necessary funds, but they're invested in some other vehicle that is yielding a significantly higher return than the new equipment is likely to produce. In such a case, however, it should be easy to borrow the money and then buy for cash rather than lease.

4. You need equipment that should be replaced frequently as technological improvements are introduced. This is one outstanding benefit of leasing.

If you are thinking of leasing, you and your tax adviser should review the leasing company's proposal. Look closely at these points:

The investment-tax credit. If the lease is properly drawn you may be able to obtain the tax credit even though the equipment remains the property of the leasing company.

Disposition of the equipment at the end of the lease term. As I mentioned earlier, to avoid problems with the I.R.S., this must be done correctly. Be skeptical if the leasing company makes the expressed or implied assumption that by the end of the lease period the equipment will have lost most of its value and should be replaced. Most dental and medical equipment has a longer life than five or eight years. A leasing company's profit comes largely from the financing of the new equipment *plus* its residual value at the end of the lease. Any meaningful comparison of leasing with some form of outright purchase must take into account a realistic salvage value.

The other conditions of the lease. Some of the conditions may be negotiable, depending on the current state of the money market. For example, will you have to pay for extra life insurance? Shop around. You may be surprised at the differences in proposals you'll get from the leasing companies.

If you decide to borrow the money to pay for your construction and equipment, read Chapter 18 on financing a building. Although this type of loan is different, the strategy and tactics involved are the same.

You'll want to convince the banker that you're a good credit risk and a good customer (or potential customer). Your letter to the bank that accompanies your formal loan application should include:

☐ the amount you want to borrow, and for how long;

☐ why you want the loan, including specific details of how you will use it;

☐ how you wish to repay the loan;

☐ a biographical sketch of yourself;

☐ your type of practice and how long you've been in practice;

☐ the competition in the area and why you believe you'll prosper;

☐ your personal financial condition and outstanding loans (even if your professional corporation is borrowing the money you'll be asked to guarantee the loan personally);

☐ a realistic projection of your earning power during the term of the loan;

☐ why granting your loan will be beneficial for the bank—include the likely level of your checking account balance and the other business you may be able to refer to the bank; and

☐ the collateral or security you can offer. This will usually be the office equipment and furniture.

Before you apply for the loan, discuss with your tax adviser what entity should buy the equipment. Some doctors who are incorporated have found it beneficial to buy the equipment as individuals or partnerships; then they lease it to their professional corporation. This arrangement may have advantages for your personal tax situation.

Be careful if the banker speaks in terms of a "discounted" or "add-on" note. This is a loan in which the interest is deducted in advance, but you must repay the face amount. Always ask if the rate quoted is the *true annual interest rate*.

The best kind of loan is one for which you are charged simple interest on the unpaid balance—at the lowest rate you can get, of course.

The length of the loan can be important. Many banks are reluctant to allow this type of loan to extend more than five to seven years. From your viewpoint, usually, the longer the better. The bank may allow you, if you're just starting in practice, to defer your payments for three or six months.

The banker may speak as if there is no alternative to repaying your loan on a monthly basis. While this is the way most consumer loans are repaid, business loans are often negotiated differently. For example, you might want to repay 5 percent of the principal every three months along with accrued interest. Thus, if your loan is for $50,000 at 14 percent for five years, every 90 days you would repay $2,500 plus interest on the unpaid balance. Paying off your loan in this way gives you the use of the money for a longer time. It may be more convenient than having to pay each month.

Don't be afraid to negotiate. The worst that the banker can do is say No to some of your requests. If you have a strong bargaining position, you may be able to get the terms you want.

III
YOUR OWN OFFICE BUILDING: HOW TO BEGIN

12

THE FEASIBILITY STUDY: IS THE PROJECT WORTHWHILE?

Your decision to erect a new building sets in motion a chain of events. It can end with you as the proud owner of an attractive, well-designed structure that is self-supporting and easily salable. It can also end with you staggering for years under a crushing financial burden as the owner of a building that cost far more than expected and has empty office suites.

The important early decisions, which in large measure determine the outcome of the project, must be based on a sound analysis of the investment. This *feasibility study* is vital if you are to have a clear grasp of the risks and rewards involved. The analysis should be prepared by someone with knowledge of:

☐ local land costs;
☐ building and site-development costs;
☐ local real-estate taxes;
☐ financing availability and sources;
☐ building operating expenses;
☐ current availability of office rental space; and
☐ competitive rental rates in the area.

Your accountant or lawyer can perform the study if one of them has the necessary real-estate background. Other experts who can also do it are a professional management consultant, or a professional real-estate consultant or appraiser. (What these experts do is presented in Chapter 3.)

Most important are the objectivity and the accuracy of the estimates used in the study. You're going to risk a lot of time and money in this project. If the analysis is faulty, you'll be taking far greater risks than you may realize. Overoptimistic projections are dangerous. They are most likely if your analyst has something to gain from a decision to proceed with the project. That's why architects, builders, and real-estate or mortgage brokers may not be the people to prepare your feasibility study. Yet they may be the only ones available to you who are capable of doing it. If you're in doubt about the results of the study, don't proceed until you verify them with a second opinion.

The figures in your study should be estimates, not of current costs and rents, but what those amounts are likely to be six months to one year in the future—at the time your building is going up. Construction costs have been increasing at a rate of at least one percent or more per month in 1980. They're likely to continue to grow with a speed that depends on the inflation rate.

TABLE 12-1*

Estimate of Cost

1.	Land	$ _____
2.	Building	_____
3.	Site improvements	_____
4.	Architect	_____
5.	Legal services	_____
6.	Professional management	_____
7.	Financing	_____
8.	Engineering	_____
9.	Appraisal	_____
10.	Building permit and licenses	_____
11.	Construction loan interest	_____
12.	Insurance	_____
13.	Contingencies	_____
14.	Total estimated cost	$ _____

*Tables 12-1 to 12-4 originally appeared in slightly different form in *Dental Management*, May 1973. Copyright by Harcourt Brace Jovanovich Inc. Reprinted by permission. All items in parentheses as well as the explanations of the tables are my interpretations.

Notes for Table 12-1

This portion of the study is important because it determines how much financing you'll need, and it affects estimates in the other tables.

Line 2. The cost of the building depends partly on who does the interior construction in the various suites. If the owners pay only for the *shell*, while each tenant pays for the electrical work, plumbing, partitions, dropped ceilings, and floor coverings in his own office, the construction cost is substantially lower than if the owners pay for this construction. A more common approach is to set up a list of interior construction allowances to be provided by the owners, based on the square-foot area of each suite. Any costs above these limits are paid by the tenants. Only the amount to be paid by the owners should be included on Line 2. If your building is a single-office structure, such as one housing a group practice, however, your analysis will include the office's entire interior construction as part of the building's costs.

Line 3. Site improvements include parking, driveways, sidewalks, exterior lighting, landscaping, and sewer and water connection.

Line 4. This fee is discussed in Chapter 4. It should be about 7 to 12 percent of the budgeted construction cost.

Line 6. Management of your property during construction is likely to be needed only if your building is large and you need someone, such as a clerk-of-the-works, at the job at all times.

Line 7. The costs of obtaining a mortgage and a construction loan, such as a mortgage broker's commission and/or points, not the interest on the loan itself.

Line 8. Engineering includes soil testing, site survey, topographical survey, planning of mechanical needs. Architect's fee may include some of these.

Line 9. The lending institution will want its appraiser to examine your site, review your plans and specifications, and estimate what the finished structure will be worth. You pay his fee.

Line 13. This category includes such items as charges for blasting to remove rock from the excavation, cost of diverting an unexpected underground stream, or special waterproofing techniques for the foundation.

TABLE 12-2
Estimate of Annual Income, Expense, and Cash Flow

Estimated rental income:

Floor no.	Rentable sq. ft.	Rental per sq. ft.	Gross income
_____	_____	_____	_____
_____	_____	_____	_____
1. Totals (1a) _____		(1b) _____	_____
2. Estimated vacancy loss (____%)			(−) _____
3. Estimated gross income			_____

Estimated operating expenses:

4. Taxes	_____	11. Scavenger service	_____
5. Insurance	_____	12. Management	_____
6. Electricity	_____	13. Legal, administrative, and accounting	_____
7. Salaries	_____		
8. Water	_____	14. Repairs and replacements	_____
9. Snow removal	_____	15. Maintenance supplies	_____
10. Service contracts	_____	16. Fuel	_____

17. Total (4-16)   (−) _____

18. Estimated operating net income (Line 3 minus Line 17)   _____

19. Mortgage principal (annual)   _____

20. Interest (annual)   _____

21. Total (19, 20)   (−) _____

22. Estimated annual surplus (Line 18 minus Line 21) (before income taxes)   _____

23. Estimated operating net income (from Line 18)   _____

24. Interest   _____

25. Depreciation   _____

26. Total (24, 25)   (−) _____

27. Taxable income   _____

28. Estimated tax   (−) _____

29. Estimated (after-tax) net annual surplus   _____

Notes for Table 12-2

Line 1a. Note the term *rentable square feet*. This is not the same as *usable square feet*, which is the space within each office. The rentable area is the building's suites plus a proportionate share of common space such as lobby, hallways, and public lavatories. The total rentable square feet, in turn, is normally about 15 to 20 percent less than the gross square-foot area of the building, for the latter also includes the outside walls plus certain interior areas not usually counted as rentable footage. There are several variations of this portion of the feasibility study. In some versions, the gross area rather than the rentable area is used in the calculations.

Line 1b. Rental per square foot can be determined by Table 12-4. This amount is subject to escalation due to increases in operating expenses, especially energy costs and changes in tax rates.

Line 2. Vacancy rate would be zero if all suites were occupied by owner-tenants. It could be 25 percent or higher if there were an abundance of office rental space in your area and you have difficulty finding tenants for the extra space in your building. A vacancy rate higher than anticipated is an important cause of losses in the operation of professional office buildings. That's why many consultants advise doctors to build structures only large enough to house the owner-tenants, but with provision for expansion.

Line 4. The tax estimate, which includes real-estate, personal-property, and payroll taxes, should take into account any possible real-es-

tate tax exemptions or reductions. Some communities offer these to encourage new commercial construction, such as professional office buildings. Payroll taxes are involved only if building is to have regular salaried maintenance employees.

Line 5. Include fire and liability insurance.

Line 6. This expense is for the building only—lobby, hallway, and exterior lighting, operation of heating system, air conditioning. Tenants should have their own electric meters.

Line 7. Salaries are for employed maintenance workers.

Line 10. This category includes boiler and air-conditioning inspection and maintenance, window washing, floor waxing.

Line 12. You need this only if your building is quite large.

Line 16. This estimate needs careful evaluation of alternative energy sources. Future costs are difficult to calculate.

Line 18. Projected operating expenses are subtracted from your estimated gross income to arrive at this figure.

Lines 19 and 20. Principal and interest payments differ each year as payments of principal increase and interest payments decrease. However, Line 21, the sum of Lines 19 and 20, remains the same each year if you have a fixed-rate mortgage (discussed Chapter 18).

Lines 22 to 29. To get the figure on Line 22, the annual debt service, that is, mortgage principal plus interest, is subtracted from the net income estimate. Repayment of principal is not strictly an expense, since it increases your equity in the

building, but it's still cash that must be paid. If your building is operated by an individual or partnership, this estimated annual surplus (Line 22) is known as the *cash flow*. It's the approximate dollar amount you might expect your building to throw off annually after all obligations are paid. If costs exceed income, your surplus turns to a deficit, and you have a *negative cash flow*. You and your partners must make up the difference.

If your building is operated as a corporation, it must pay taxes on this surplus. The corporation's cash flow is the *after-tax* net annual surplus on Line 29. This is obtained by subtracting mortgage interest and depreciation estimates, which are tax-deductible items, from the estimated operating net income (Line 18) to obtain the taxable income. After the appropriate corporate tax is subtracted, the remainder is the estimated net surplus for a corporation.

The figure you enter on Line 25 for depreciation depends on how your accountant calculates it. There are several formulas used to calculate accelerated depreciation. In addition, your accountant may use *component depreciation*, in which different parts of the project are assigned different useful life expectancies for purposes of depreciation.

You can't really calculate an after-tax surplus for a partnership because partnerships don't pay taxes. Each partner reports his share of the partnership's cash flow (minus depreciation) on his own income-tax return. Usually, at least in the early years of a building, this shows as a substantial loss that helps to offset your ordinary income.

TABLE 12-3

Estimate of Capital Requirement

1. Total project cost
   (from Table 12-1, Line 14)   _____

2. a) any portion of land not
      allocable to project _____

   b) Any portion of site
      improvements not allocable
      to project _____

   Total of a and b   (−) _____

3. Estimated net project cost   _____

4. Estimated mortgage obtainable (−) _____

5. Balance (Line 3 minus Line 4)   _____

6. Land and site improvements not
   allocable to project   (+) _____

7. Estimated capital required
   (Line 5 plus Line 6)   _____

Notes for Table 12-3

Line 2. These items are pertinent only if you have to buy more land than you need for the building plus the drives and parking area. The cost of the extra land and any site improvements on it are usually not considered part of the building project when the mortgage is being considered. That is why they are deducted from the project cost for the purposes of estimating the mortgage obtainable, but added back (Line 6) when the capital requirement (cash needed) is calculated.

Line 3. The amount on which your mortgage is based.

Line 7. This is the dollar amount you and your partners have to provide to get the structure built. It may or may not include the cost of interior construction in the owner-tenants' individual offices. It doesn't include equipping or furnishing individual offices. Even if your estimates are accurate, it's prudent to add 10 to 20 percent for contingencies in construction.

Tables 12-1 to 12-4 show the kinds of estimates needed and how they are handled in a feasibility study. Note that some information has to be juggled back and forth between the tables before final estimates can be arrived at.

Keep in mind that the numbers to be used can be only estimates, not firm figures, and that your expert may do the analysis on a somewhat different form than the tables shown; there's nothing rigid about any of it. Whatever form your expert uses, you'll get some valuable bottom-line insights.

Tables 12-3 and 12-4, for example, are intended to produce two important figures: *capital required*—how much you will have to invest—and *rental rate*—how much you will have to charge in rent per rentable square foot.

These are both crucial numbers because they may determine whether your project should proceed. If the capital required is too great for you to handle alone, you'll have to add partners to help spread the load or you'll have to abandon the venture. If the rental rate arrived at is significantly higher than the existing rents in the area, you may have empty suites for a long time. If you try to keep your rents below the level indicated by the study, you may find that your building is not self-supporting (it has a *negative cash flow)*. You and your partners will then have to make up this deficit each year.

Examine the project separately as an investor and as a future tenant in the building. As a tenant, you'll want the space you need at a reasonable rent. As an investor, you'll look for a higher return on your investment compared with other ways you can invest your money. The investment return in Table 12-4, line 3, is calculated as a percentage of capital invested (some analysts may calculate it as a percentage of net project cost). Unless you can achieve a satisfactory return, your building won't be a good investment in comparison with other ways you can invest your money.

Your total yield will be the annual cash flow—the amount referred to as investment yield in Table 12-4, plus the tax-sheltering effect of depreciation, plus the increase in your equity as the mortgage is paid off (assuming that the building's value appreciates). If you're considering the building primarily as an investment, this total yield should be well above the inflation rate.

Don't be surprised if the feasibility study suggests that there may be little or no cash flow, or even a negative cash flow. Many medical buildings are not highly profitable investments. You may decide to drop the whole idea and find another approach to setting up an office. Or you may resolve to go ahead, even though the building won't be an outstanding investment. Owning your own building may be the only way to get the office you need without the possibility of exorbitant rent increases every few years.

The feasibility study, remember, is an attempt to anticipate what's in store for you if you put up a new building. If the analysis is done with realistic numbers, you'll at least be entering the deal with your eyes open.

If the feasibility analysis seems to show that your plan to erect a professional office building is worthwhile, your next steps should be to:
☐ find your architect (Chapter 4);
☐ start your search for possible sites (Chapter 14);
☐ begin inquiries about financing (Chapter 18); and
☐ start looking for partners if you need them (Chapter 13).

TABLE 12-4

Estimate of Rental Rate Requirement

1. Total estimated operating expenses (Table 12-2, Line 17) _____

2. (Debt service) (Table 12-2, Line 21) _____

3. Investment yield (___% of capital to be invested) (Table 12-3, Line 7) _____

4. Total Lines 1, 2, and 3 _____

5. Adjustment for estimated vacancy loss (___% of Line 4) _____

6. Estimated gross rental income requirement (Line 4 plus Line 5) _____

7. Estimated rental rate required: annual per square foot (Line 6 divided by net rentable square feet in building, Table 12-2, Line 1a) _____

Notes for Table 12-4

Line 3. This figure should be competitive with what a similar investment would earn elsewhere *if* investment income is your principal goal.
Line 5. Vacancy rate will be zero if only owner-tenants occupy the building. Otherwise, vacancy rate could be high.

13
WORKING WITH PARTNERS

There is no aspect of professional office building construction more likely to ruin your disposition and your digestion than the unsound choice of partners.

The doctor who starts a building project, when he is looking for partners, is typically preoccupied with numbers more than with other factors. A willingness to advance the money may be all that is needed for admission to the partnership. If partners aren't more carefully chosen, problems often develop later. Here are some of them:

1. Doctors of widely differing ages may have quite different investment and retirement goals which can affect the tax treatment of the project.

2. The personalities of some doctors may adversely affect the group. Some doctors in solo practice are unaccustomed to the give-and-take of working with others. Each may expect his every wish to be fulfilled just as it always was in his own office.

3. More than one doctor may feel that because of some prior experience he should be the one to lead the project.

4. Once the enthusiasm and euphoria marking the start of the project have subsided, the doctors find they disagree on what kind of building they want.

5. A doctor's spouse, especially one with training in architecture or design, can be a source of serious difficulty by attempting to impose ideas of design or decoration on the group.

6. A doctor or group of doctors who plan to use a large portion of the building for their own offices may feel that their influence in decision making should be in proportion to the area they'll occupy.

You can prevent some of these problems if you follow up on these points:

If you're the originator and leader of the project: Start looking for partners only *after* your feasibility study has been performed and a proposal is in writing.

This should include realistic projections of the time, costs, risks, and benefits of being an owner-tenant in your building.

The proposal should also outline clearly the powers, responsibilities, and rewards of the governing partner (organizer) or partners. This might be yourself and perhaps one deputy. It should be clearly understood at the outset of the project that its supervision must be in the hands of only one or two people if the too-many-cooks syndrome is to be avoided. Continuity of decision making is vital. The partnership agreement, discussed below, should spell out these points in detail.

Look for partners who are similar to yourself in age, in economic status, and in background. The more homogeneous the group is, the easier it should be to draw up a partnership agreement that satisfies the needs of all partners. However, an experienced attorney can usually make provision for the varying goals of doctors in different age brackets.

You'll probably have fewer headaches if you limit your group to doctors who will occupy space in the building. While it's true that the more partners there are, the less is the risk for each, it also means that the chances of disagreements are greatly increased.

Don't plan to build extra space unless you are certain that additional suites will be easy to rent. Many doctors believe that building space for rental is a good way to increase the building's income. But many have found out too late that construction of professional office space for profit is best left to the real-estate professionals. Negotiating leases, responding to the complaints of tenants, and trying to fill vacant suites are problems you can do without.

If you're invited to become a partner: You may have decided that you need a new office, but are you sure that the role of owner-tenant is best for you? Have you considered all the other alternatives discussed in Chapter 2?

Do you have confidence in the originator of the project? Is this confidence based on his air of assurance and his being a "nice guy," or is it based on his willingness and ability to provide you with figures and facts that you can verify independently? And you *should* verify them independently.

Do you have enough rapport with the governing partner and with the group to make likely the equitable solution of disputes? If there are any difficult individuals who appear abrasive or rigid now, how will they be later if unexpected problems and costs develop?

Are you willing to go along with the governing partner even if your own pet design ideas or your favorite builder are turned down?

Have the full details of the building proposal and the partnership arrangement been given to you, in writing, before you are asked to sign anything or to advance any money? Be especially wary if, in response to your request for details, you get a casual, "Don't worry, Joe. We'll work those things out later."

THE PARTNERSHIP AGREEMENT

Whether you're the originator of the project or have been invited by the organizer to join, you and everyone else in the partnership will benefit by having a written agreement, prepared by an experienced attorney, before any firm decisions are made. This agreement should be carefully reviewed by each member separately with his own lawyer and financial adviser. Following are some of the areas that should be covered by the agreement:

1. Is the group to operate as a partnership or as a corporation? The partnership mode is often better, at least in the early years of building ownership, from a tax standpoint, but with our ever-changing tax structure you'd better get your accountant's advice before deciding. You might ask, too, about operating the building as a condominium.

2. How much latitude is to be given to the project organizer in decision making? Has he been given signatory powers for contracts and other documents? Has a "hold-harmless" clause been inserted to protect him if the project sours?

3. What remuneration is to be given to the project organizer for his extra efforts and time in the group's behalf? He will have to take hundreds—yes, hundreds—of hours from his practice and family. The reward could be an additional equity percentage or it might take some other form.

4. How are the partners to vote when decisions are to be made? Is it to be one person, one vote or is voting to be weighted, based on the percentage of equity that each one has in the project? Is the governing partner to have more than one vote?

5. When the group votes on any matter, how great a majority will be needed to carry a motion? Unanimity? Three-fourths? Two-thirds? A simple majority? This must be clear. If you are the governing partner, will you be able to face the possibility that you could be outvoted? Now is the time—before it is too late—to consider how to handle such a problem.

6. How much money is each partner to put up and when must it be paid?

7. How are unexpected costs to be covered? What penalty is to be exacted if a partner is unable to meet an emergency call for capital? If any partner does not contribute his share on time, he might be required to pay a very high rate of interest—perhaps 1.5 times the prime rate—to the partner who advances the money for him until he puts up the necessary cash.

8. How and when are profits or losses to be allocated once the building is in use? Some groups decide to retain all profits, if any, for a number of years rather than to distribute them to the members.

9. What will be each owner-tenant's rights and responsibilities in the cost of design and construction of his own offices? Where is the boundary between what the building partnership should provide and what the doctor should be expected to pay for himself? For example, for each 1,000 square feet of office space, an owner-tenant might be entitled to 100 lineal feet of partitions, six doors, one three-ton air-conditioning unit, and 40 feet of ductwork. Similar suite-development allowances should be set up for electrical, lighting, plumbing, and other needs. Any amounts over the allowances would then have to be paid by the owner-tenant. If you decide on this approach, remember that these allowances should be included in your feasibility study as part of the construction cost (see Table 12-1, Line 2).

A comparable arrangement should be provided for design services. The building architect's contract should cover the building shell, but design services for each doctor are best handled separately. Since doctors in different specialties have dissimilar needs, the architect's services for planning partitions, casework, and mechanical details can be compensated for on an hourly or a negotiated fee basis.

10. What will be expected of each owner-tenant after the building is occupied? Responsibility for management chores, such as changing light bulbs, cleaning lobby and halls, and snow plowing, should in theory be rotated among the owner-tenants if the building isn't large enough to warrant a full-time manager. But it rarely works out that way. Frequently one partner, because of inclination or experience, becomes the manager, and he should be compensated for his services.

11. When and how can a member withdraw from the group? Apart from death, the most frequently permitted reasons are permanent disability, military service, or retirement at a particular age. In special circumstances, the group could vote to permit withdrawal for other reasons.

Here are some ways to protect the remaining partners against serious financial burdens.

Each owner-tenant signs a lease with a term as long as the term of the mortgage. This assures the building of continuing income for mortgage payments.

If a doctor in solo practice dies or becomes disabled, his lease might be canceled when his estate pays a penalty to the partnership of three to five months of rent. Of course, if the doctor who died was part of a group practice, the lease would not be affected.

To deter any partner from withdrawing early, you may specify that no withdrawals are permitted during the first three or four years. If a partner must leave during this time, he'd recoup only a small percentage of his investment.

Life insurance can be used by the partnership to buy out the equity of a deceased partner. But since the premiums may be high for older partners, and since they are not deductible, it's good to look for other alternatives. In the first years of the building's use, each partner's equity is relatively small if you've gotten the largest possible mortgage. It may be feasible, through additional contributions by the other partners, to buy out the interest of a partner who died. Later on, when larger sums are involved, it may make sense to refinance the building to get the necessary dollars.

12. How is a departing member's share to be valued? Appraised market value is fairer than book value. Over how long a period is it to be paid? The formula often used is 10 to 25 percent in cash, with the balance as notes payable over a three- to seven-year period.

13. How can a new owner-tenant be added to the group?

14. Under what circumstances can a member be expelled from the partnership? These might include conviction for criminal activities that endanger the group's welfare.

15. What happens if a few partners wish to withdraw simultaneously? This could happen if the neighborhood deteriorates or if several owners who are at or above retirement age decide to draw out their equity and retire at the same time. How is the load on the remaining partners to be managed?

A particularly sticky situation is the breakup of a group practice in a multioffice building. If the doctors in the group are also part owners of the building, there can be increased friction—or worse—in the management of the building. Some kind of buy-out arrangement should be planned for this kind of problem.

16. What is to be the group's policy on engaging the services of relatives of partners? "My brother's a lawyer. He can draw up our partnership agreement and contracts at a minimum fee." "My cousin can get us carpeting for the lobby at his wholesale cost." "My wife's uncle is in the air-conditioning business. He'll do our whole building at a terrific price!"

The temptation to save money in this way is strong. It seems at first glance that a relative or spouse will have the partnership's best interests at heart. It often does happen that way, but it's so easy for things to turn sour.

Suppose that Dr. A's brother, the lawyer, forgets an important point in the contract with the builder and you suffer a loss as a result. Will Dr. A be a party to a suit against his own brother for negligence?

Will Dr. B's cousin, who provides the carpeting for the lobby at wholesale cost, be in a hurry to replace the section that wasn't installed right initially?

What do you know about the competence of Dr. C's wife's uncle, the air-conditioning man? Will Dr. C be comfortable if you have to hold back the final payment because the system is not properly balanced?

A safe approach to this problem is to utilize your spouse's talents and your relatives' services in *your own office* to whatever extent you wish. But for the building itself and for equipping and decorating the common areas, deal with outsiders. You'll probably save yourself needless irritation.

Although many of the points in this chapter may seem remote, they are all serious problems. If you ignore them now, they may haunt you later.

14
THE SITE ANALYSIS: IS THIS THE RIGHT SPOT?

Knowledgeable real-estate investors consider the location of a property its most important feature. To you, the future owner of a professional building, a good location means easy access for patients, attractiveness to other doctor-tenants, and resale possibilities. Most practice-management consultants agree that the closer an office building is to a hospital, the more attractive it is to physicians. Since they are one of your chief sources of tenants and of likely future buyers of the building, this proximity is very important.

Get a street map of the community. With the hospital as its center draw a circle whose radius is a 10-minute drive from the center. Within this circle is the most desirable location for your building. In congested areas, this may be only two to three miles, while in towns where traffic is relatively light, the radius could be as much as eight to 10 miles. A local realtor should be able to show you the available sites within the circle.

Look first for land within a few blocks of the hospital, and then farther away. If the hospital owns a substantial amount of open land, you might consider leasing land from it for your building. If the hospital does have vacant land, however, first find out if it has plans to use it for a doctors' office building that would compete for tenants with the building you're planning to put up.

You'll be looking for property that is not only in a good location, but is priced right. When you've narrowed your choice to one or a few properties, call in your architect. With your help, he should perform the study described below before you agree to the purchase.

The seller may press you for a decision. Don't let yourself be rushed. You can buy an option, which will give you time to complete your investigation. A 30- or 60-day option on a property may cost several hundred dollars. It's not refundable if you turn down the purchase, but by giving you time to study the deal carefully it can save you from making a serious mistake.

The careful evaluation of a piece of property as a site for your building is known as *site analysis.* Its purpose is to find out if the site is suitable for building and, if so, to determine how to use the land to its best advantage. If the analysis is done well it can tell you, long before a shovelful of earth is moved and even before the building is designed, approximately what expenses you'll face for *site development.* Preparing the land for your building can cost a great deal of money; it's better not to be caught unaware.

A well-informed builder or architect can tell you, without seeing a property, the likely construction costs per square foot of building in your area. But he would hesitate to even guess at the cost of site work without studying the lot. Also, a lending institution usually bases its mortgage commitment primarily on the building itself, not on the cost of preparing the site for the structure. If there are major unplanned-for costs for site work, you may have to pay for them as "extras" during construction, when most of your funds are committed to other aspects of the project.

For all these reasons, site analysis is one of the most important steps in the sequence leading to erection of your building. Here are some of the more important points you and your architect will study:

Zoning. Does the local zoning code permit your type of building on this site? Don't take the broker's word for it. Go to the municipal building or zoning department office and ask to see a current zoning map of the area. Try to get a photocopy for your records. The clerk can explain what the map symbols mean. If the site is not presently zoned for office buildings, you must make your purchase contingent on getting a variance. Zoning and other local restrictions are discussed in more detail in Chapter 15.

Size. Is the property large enough for the structure you want, for enough parking spaces, and for landscaping, plus room for future expansion? To get an idea of how many parking spaces are needed, add together the number of doctors, assistants—full- and part-time—and patients likely to be treated and waiting at the busiest time of the week. Allow for one car per person. One parking space per 100 square feet of usable office space should be more than adequate unless there is a high-volume practice in the building. If street parking is permitted, less on-site space is needed. Remember, however, that street parking regulations can change overnight.

Visual impact. What kind of appearance will a building have on this site? Does it belong in this neighborhood? Will you be proud to drive up to it? Will its presence arouse neighborhood antagonism? Your architect has to consider not only this, but how the building must be oriented on the lot, where the entry should be in relation to the environment, and how pedestrians and cars will move around the building.

Access. Are the local street arrangements and traffic flow such that patients can easily reach your office? Will it be safe and convenient for them to turn into and out of your parking area?

Is the site easily accessible by public transportation? With the threat of energy shortages a constant feature of our lives today, patients may now and then have to travel by this means.

Topography. What kind of surface does the lot have? Is it flat? Sloped? Banked? Will *cuts* and/or *fills* be needed? A cut is the removal of earth from high points; a fill is the addition of soil to low areas. Are there rock outcroppings that have to be removed? Is there a pond or creek that must be drained or diverted? Does adjoining property drain into the one you're considering?

Subsurface features. Is there underground water? Rock? Does the soil have adequate bearing capacity for the projected size of your building? Will the building need special supports, such as piles or extra foundations? Does the soil have suitable permeability for drainage? If not, your building could be an island in a lake after heavy rains.

To find out about these and other characteristics of the earth, the architect may have to call in a soils engineer to make test borings at various parts of the property.

Vegetation. Trees and shrubs are important on a property, not only because of their appearance, but because their roots firmly hold the soil in sloping areas, they reduce erosion and absorb water, the oxygen they produce improves the environment, and trees serve as sound and wind barriers.

Are there trees or shrubs on the property that are worth saving? Are there large trees that will be expensive to remove now or later? Even though a tree is not in the part of the property to be excavated for the building, its root structure may be so damaged by changes around it that it may die within a year or two and require removal. There is an enormous variation in the susceptibility of trees to the change in the grade around them. Maples may die when the grade around them is changed less than six inches, yet I have some locust trees that survived and even thrived after eight feet of earth was dumped around their trunks.

Water, sanitary sewers, and storm sewers. Are the existing utilities adequate to service your building? Where are they in relation to the proposed location of the building on the site? Digging trenches for burying pipes can cost many dollars per running foot. You'll want to keep them to a minimum. How deep are the storm sewers? Are they large enough to handle the runoff from your property? Are they deep enough underground to accept drainage pipes running from around your foundation?

Who supplies water, the municipality or a private company? Is it permitted to use water to cool an air-conditioning unit? Is pressure adequate? Will taste, color, or turbidity require special filters? Are the sanitary sewers capable of handling the sewage flow from your building? You can get answers to many of these questions at the building inspector's or the municipal engineer's office. There, too, if there are no sanitary sewers, you or your architect can find out about any septic-system requirements. Ask, also, if there are special regulations concerning driveways, curbs, and sidewalks and hook-ups to utility lines.

Energy. Is adequate electric power available at the voltages you'll need? Some heavy equipment works most economically on three-phase current at 230 volts. Is this available? Is natural gas available for heating your building, or must you rely on oil deliveries? The local utility company will provide answers to these questions.

Telephones. Is there adequate telephone service available? Can push-button phones be used instead of dial phones? Ask the phone company.

Legal considerations. Your attorney will have to check for troublesome inclusions in the owner's deed, such as covenants, easements, or other restrictions. Local ordinances and master plans must also be examined for possible problems. These are considered in Chapter 15.

Taxes. The local assessor can provide information on any pending changes in methods of assessment or taxation in the area. Equally important, does the community offer tax abatements or concessions to new commercial buildings?

When the site analysis is completed, you and your architect should have a good idea of whether this is the right place for your building. He should also be able to suggest the type of building suitable for the site, its location and its orientation on the property, as well as the costs of the site work needed to prepare the land for your building.

15
ZONING: WILL YOUR BUILDING BE PERMITTED?

A little historical background may help us to understand what zoning is and why it is so unpredictable. In the 19th century, as factories sprouted everywhere in American towns and cities, they often produced unsightly and smelly by-products. Many communities started to restrict the areas where such industry could develop, in order to keep factories out of residential areas. The legal justification for this "zoning" was that the towns were protecting their citizens from public nuisances. But, in so doing, the municipalities were setting precedents establishing the right of the community to tell property owners how their land could and could not be used.

In the 1920s, came the systematic division of communities into zones where only certain types of uses were permitted, such as residential, commercial, or industrial. The principal underlying motivation behind most early zoning laws was to protect the owners of single-family homes from real or perceived threats to the value of their property.

More recently, many communities have developed master plans, schemes drawn up by professional planners to guide the orderly growth of the area. The master plan suggests what would be the most appropriate use for land in each part of the community. It doesn't have legal standing, but the local authorities are likely to follow it when they rule on zoning ordinances.

Many of the state laws that permit local zoning ordinances are written in broad terms, consequently, local laws are often not uniform from one town to another. Even if the laws in adjoining towns are similar, interpretations by local officials may differ. That's why zoning and how it's enforced can be unpredictable, arbitrary, and infuriating.

Local zoning ordinances generally are divided into two broad categories called *use requirements* and *bulk requirements.*

The town map is zoned into many different districts—residential, professional office, laboratory-office, commercial, and industrial, to name a few. The text and the tables accompanying the map specify the *uses* allowed for land in each zone.

Bulk requirements, the second part of the zoning law, specify for each zone such things as the maximum height allowed for a building, how far back from the street and from the property lines the building must be placed, and how many parking spaces must be provided. For example, a commonly used parking requirement is one on-site parking space for each 100 or 200 square feet of building area.

To understand better how zoning works, let's look at two possible scenarios. In one, the site you select for your building is, fortunately, in a zone where such use is permitted. In the second, the lot, which looks like the ideal location for your building, is in a zone in which that kind of construction is not allowed.

SCENARIO #1

Your architect goes to the office of the *building inspector,* the local official charged with enforcing the zoning and building laws. He learns that the site you've picked is in a zone called "Professional Offices." So far, so good. He now looks at the bulk requirements in the zoning act and finds that your lot is large enough for a building of the size you want to erect. You'll be able to meet the height and the setback restrictions (the required distances from the property lines), and you'll have room for more than enough parking. Looks like clear sailing.

Assuming that your feasibility study and the rest of your site analysis are favorable and the price is right, you buy the land, and your architect proceeds with his drawings. One of the first will be the *site plan,* which will show the size and location of the building on the lot as well as driveways and parking areas. He'll submit this plan, along with other details of the proposed building, to the building inspector and the local *planning board.*

This board has the responsibility for *site-plan review* of each new construction project. It examines the site plan and accompanying data to be sure that your building conforms in all respects to the zoning law. The planning board calls in its technical advisers (staff members or consultants) for opinions on different aspects of the project. These may include the town engineer, the building inspector, the town planner, the fire commissioner, and possibly others. All of them report back to the planning board about the impact of the new building on the community's traffic flow, drainage, sewer capacity, and other factors.

Another group that may be involved is the *architectural review board* (A.R.B.). The planning board asks its opinion about your new building. The A.R.B. is interested in what its appearance and color are to be and in the materials your architect plans to use. The A.R.B.'s recommendations relate to the suitability of the design for that neighborhood. If your project involves restoring an old building in a historic district, the A.R.B. will want to know whether and how your renovation will change the building's appearance. The A.R.B. may or may not have official veto power over your project, but its comments are given serious consideration by the planning board.

Once the planning board has received the reports of its experts and is satisfied that there are no major problems, it issues a *site-plan approval*, which says to the building inspector, in effect, "This project looks O.K. Let it go ahead, but make sure that the following conditions are met." Then it may list changes that your architect will have to make in the plans before the inspector issues a *building permit*, the official permission to begin construction.

Notice that even though your proposed building meets all of the community's zoning requirements, it may take a great deal of time in getting the project past the various agencies and boards. Some officials create long delays in settling drainage problems, for example, or arrangement of driveways, and require that the proposal be bounced back and forth among different groups for months before final approval is granted. This tactic is often used when there is local opposition to the building, even though it's in a proper zone.

One method that can expedite the process, assuming that all the local officials are acting in good faith, is for your architect to meet with the town's engineer, planner, building inspector and other technical experts *before* submitting the site plan to the planning board. He can explain the project in an informal session. They, in turn, will point out what must be done to obtain their approval. In that way, by the time the planning board sees the proposal, it will be in a form that will meet few objections—you hope!—and your construction can begin.

SCENARIO #2

This time you're not so lucky. You or your architect looks at the zoning map and you find that your site is in a zone labeled "Residential, One- and Two-Family Dwellings." No professional office buildings are allowed. What should you do? Abandon the project or try to get it approved?

There is no single answer to that question. You have to find out how similar problems have been resolved in that community. Local officials and real-estate people can probably tell you. But even if there are precedents that seem to indicate that you can ultimately get permission to build, you may have to go through a long, long wait.

One approach is to seek a *change of zone.* For example, if your lot is in a residential zone, and the property next door is in a commercial zone, you might have a chance to get the town board (or whatever the local legislative body is called) to change your property to commercial zoning. You might get your change of zone, too, if the zoning you want coincides with the community's master plan. Or the legislative body might even be willing to amend the zoning statute to permit your proposed use without changing the zone your property is in. Much depends on the circumstances and the neighbors' support or opposition to the idea. Note that only the local legislative body is empowered to change a zone or create new zones.

If this method fails, another agency now gets into the act: the zoning board of appeals (often known just as the zoning board or the Z.B.A.). This agency interprets the zoning ordinance. It can permit the use of property in ways that are contrary to the zoning law. Such permission is called a *variance.* The Z.B.A.

grants a variance when it's satisfied that the change is in the best interests of the community or that enforcement of the existing law is causing undue hardship to the owner of the property.

Usually, after notification is sent to nearby property owners, a public hearing is held on the question. This experience can be—as ours was—a pleasant exposure to municipal self-government, following which the request is approved. It can also be a harrowing inquisition that ends with a resounding No. It's hard to predict what kind of reception you'll receive.

You may strengthen your chance for success if you engage a local attorney to represent you at the hearing, one who "knows the ropes" in the community. You and your attorney must be prepared with a thorough knowledge of the existing local zoning ordinance, the ways in which your project differs from it, the precedents for your variance, and arguments to counter any likely opposition. Do your homework carefully. It would help, too, to have your architect there with preliminary plans or a model to show how your building will enhance the area.

The zoning variance you should ask for is the one that will give you latitude for the future. Ask for a change, for example, in a residential zone to permit commercial use or professional offices, not just to allow only medical or only dental offices. You may want to rent space later to a lawyer or to an accountant. Also, when you sell your building, you don't want to have to apply for a new variance if the buyer is in a different profession.

Stay cool. These hearings often become emotionally charged. If the board rules against your request, your attorney may cite favorable decisions in similar cases in other parts of the state. If the board decides, however, that those rulings don't apply in your case, your only recourse is to appeal to the courts. Unless there's a great amount at stake, you'll probably abandon the project before going that route.

Courts are frequently reluctant to superimpose their judgment over that of the municipality. Even if you win in court—usually at great cost in time and money—the local authorities may still throw enough other obstacles in your path to prevent your building from ever going up. So if the Z.B.A. turns you down, find a new location.

If your request for a variance is approved by the zoning board, you'll then have to go through all of the steps outlined above in Scenario #1 before construction of your building can begin.

OTHER GOVERNMENT REGULATIONS

Zoning isn't the only way in which the local government will affect your building. Among other influences are *building codes*, *health codes*, *standards*, *ordinances*, *easements*, and *covenants*. Let's look at each one:

Building codes are regulations that govern the materials and methods of construction to protect the safety, health, and welfare of the occupants of the building. Sometimes codes are applicable statewide, but a community's own local code may be more stringent than the state's. Compliance with the code is the architect's and the contractor's responsibility. Your architect has to know, in advance, of any special requirements, such as fire regulations that require sprinklers or other equipment. These can affect his design and can substantially increase the cost of your building. The local building agency is the source for this information.

Health codes are state, county, or local ordinances that, like building codes, are intended to protect the public from illness or injury. A health-code regulation that might affect your new office, for example, is one that requires radiation shielding in the walls that surround X-ray equipment. The local health officer or building inspector can tell you or your architect if there are any special local requirements.

Standards and ordinances govern such things as sizes, weights, and distances of items to be built, such as the width of sidewalks, height of curbs, and thickness of road blacktop. Your architect and contractor have the responsibility for complying with these.

The last two items, easements and covenants, might better be called *deed restrictions* rather than local government regulations. But since they can impede your project in ways similar to local codes, they are discussed here.

An **easement** is permission granted by an owner of a piece of property to the community, to a utility, or to some individual(s) to pass through or over or under the land. Examples might be an easement to a town to permit a "right-of-way" for road building or sewer construction or to a utility to allow erection of power transmission lines. Easements are recorded in the seller's deed or in his title-insurance policy, which should be read by your lawyer.

A **covenant** is an agreement by a property owner or group of owners that their land will be used in only certain specified ways. It's a sort of private zoning arrangement, which, like an easement, is recorded in the deed and title-insurance policy. Some covenants, such as those that restrict sale of the property to particular ethnic groups, are not legally enforceable, but others could prevent your building from ever going up. Your lawyer must find out if any such covenants exist.

Now that you're aware of the time-consuming, frustrating red tape that can be involved in these encounters with local government, are you still sure that you want to build?

16

NEGOTIATING FOR THE LAND

If your site analysis indicates that you've found the right property and if local, governmental, and legal restrictions present no problems, you are ready to buy your land.

Negotiation has been described as a meeting of minds without a knocking together of heads. It's a contest in which the adversary with the better bargaining position and/or horse-trading skill can get the terms he wants.

Circumstances vary so widely that I can't offer specific suggestions in this area. Your hand in negotiating depends a great deal on the condition of the real-estate market in the area at the time you're looking to buy.

From your feasibility study you should have a good idea of your upper price limit for land. Any substantial excess the seller demands for the land reduces its desirability.

17
CHOOSING THE BUILDER: CONVENTIONAL OR TURNKEY

There are two basic choices open to you as you consider how to get your building constructed:

The conventional approach, sometimes called *stick-and-nail* construction, involves engaging an architect to design your building and then soliciting bids from several general contractors. When one builder is selected, he engages subcontractors. (Some of the work may be done for you separately by contractors whom you engage yourself. Examples of these are the interior designer, painter, paperhanger, and alarm installer.) The architect usually observes construction as it progresses and verifies that the work is being done properly.

This is the method my colleague and I used when we renovated an old house and added a large new wing to it. It has the virtue of being familiar to everyone in the construction industry. It permits close and constant communication among the doctor, the architect, and the builder throughout all the stages of planning and construction.

The turnkey or "package" approach. A number of large companies, based in different parts of the country, would agree to undertake the entire job for you, including all design work. The expression *turnkey* is meant to indicate that you have only to turn the key in the lock and walk into your completed building and office. The building company proposes to do everything. It offers:

☐ help in finding a site;

☐ help in obtaining financing;

- [ ] architectural services (by their architects);
- [ ] engineering services;
- [ ] general contracting for complete construction and preparation of individual offices to receive your specialized equipment;
- [ ] interior design;
- [ ] decorating; and
- [ ] furnishing and cabinet installation.

The last three items are sometimes optional extras and not part of the basic construction package.

Turnkey builders claim these advantages for their concept:

Experience. They are well acquainted with the needs of most doctors in terms of such things as site analysis, building design, traffic flow, room size, quality of materials, and parking requirements.

Inexpensive preliminary planning. Some of the companies offer preliminary planning services at little or no cost. If you don't approve these plans you need not proceed any further.

One-stop shopping. The doctor has only one entity with which to negotiate. Once the contract is signed, the builder takes full responsibility for seeing the entire project through to completion.

Guaranteed price. The contract with the builder usually stipulates a firm price that cannot be increased unless the doctor decides later to change the plans.

Possible lower cost. Some of the builders claim economies of 10 to 20 percent below the cost of conventional construction. They base this on their familiarity with special techniques of construction, on their efficiency, and in some cases on the prefabrication of sections of the building in their own assembly plants. These prefinished modules are trucked to the building site and hoisted into position on a previously constructed foundation.

Guaranteed completion date. The contract usually contains a firm date when the doctor can move in, but this may have to be altered because of problems beyond the builder's control.

Many purported benefits of the turnkey concept can be matched by local architects and builders who are experienced in construction of professional office space. You can get inexpensive preliminary planning, guaranteed price, and guaranteed completion date from conventional sources if you look and negotiate hard enough.

Whether your building is done by the conventional approach or by a turnkey builder, a guaranteed price is meaningful only if no changes are necessary once the final plans are drawn. As you'll see in Chapters 35 and 52, changes and additions are costly no matter who is doing the job.

Similarly, any guaranteed completion date may be meaningless and unenforceable. Turnkey builders send their own supervisory personnel to the site and utilize local suppliers and labor for much of the work. Their job supervisor may be experienced in avoiding construction bottlenecks, but weather conditions, strikes, and delivery delays can still occur.

The lower costs attributable to the prefabricated construction and/or modular assembly used by some turnkey builders is achieved at the expense of originality of design.

Negotiation with only one entity is an advantage, but it also means relying on a distant organization for day-to-day communication before and after construction and for the enforcement of guarantees.

If you think the turnkey concept may be for you, here are a few suggestions:

1. Request literature from several such companies, not just one (a list of names and addresses can be found at the end of this chapter). Get from them the names and addresses of doctors for whom they've put up buildings. Drop from consideration any company that does not supply such a list.

2. Go to see as many of the buildings as you can get to and talk with the owners. Did the building fulfill their expectations? Did they consider the basic cost and the cost of "extras" reasonable? Was the company easy to work with? Did the company honor its warranties? Would they build again with the turnkey method? With this company?

Ask yourself how well the building fits its site. Its neighborhood. Does the quality of the work look good to you?

3. Get your own consultant. You may feel more comfortable when contracting with a turnkey builder if you have an independent architect, builder, or engineer who will serve as your consultant, accompany you to the builder's already constructed buildings to check the quality of the work, examine the plans drawn by the company's architect for possible problems, and visit your job with you during construction to spot errors or oversights.

Remember, however, to keep your own expert's comments in proper perspective. He could make unjustified critical comments to justify his fee.

4. Go through this book, making your own lists of systems and items to be included. You'll want to get everything possible into those final plans to avoid extras later.

5. Decide on your equipment before your final plans are completed. The builder will want to know exactly where each special plumbing and electrical line is to be placed, particularly if major parts of the building are to be prefabricated. Not having this information early enough in the planning process results in extra charges later.

I can't say which of the two approaches to building construction would be better for you. Each has satisfied and dissatisfied doctors. You'll have to make your decision based on the experiences of doctor friends, on your investigation of track records, and on your own gut feelings.

A few of the nationally known turnkey builders are listed here. Inclusion in the list does not imply endorsement.

American Medical Buildings
735 North Water Street
Milwaukee, Wis. 53202

BBC Health Care
1130 Hampton Avenue
St. Louis, Mo. 63169

Marshall Erdman & Associates
5117 University Avenue
Madison, Wis. 53705

Nationwide Medical-Dental Building Corp.
797 Market Street
Oregon, Wis. 53575

Professional Office Buildings
170 Ruggle Street
Fond du Lac, Wis. 54935

18
FINANCING THE BUILDING

Bankers' business is to earn money with minimum risk. As obvious as this sounds, you should keep this constantly in mind while you arrange the financing of your building. Your objective will likely be to borrow the greatest amount of money at the lowest interest rate for the longest period of time. You must convince the banker that he'll earn money safely for his bank by doing business with you on terms acceptable to you.

SPEAKING THE BANKER'S LANGUAGE

Dr. Hudson calls a local bank and asks to speak to Mr. Long, the commercial loan officer. He tells the bank officer of his proposed small professional building. The estimated completed value of the property will be about $500,000. He asks Mr. Long if the bank would like to consider financing such a project. The banker shows interest. Hudson asks what sort of terms he might expect. Long says, "We might consider 70 percent for 15 years at 14 and three." Do you know what he means?

Just as we have our professional jargon, the banker has his, and it may vary in different parts of the country. If we include all the words the banker left out of his cryptic reply, it would be something like this: "We might consider lending you 70 percent of the value of your completed building plus the land, as estimated by our appraiser, for a term of 15 years at an interest rate of 14 percent plus three points, assuming that we find you to be an acceptable risk."

When the banker tells you he will consider a 70 percent loan, he's being cautious. The lower the percentage of full value he lends you, the safer is the loan. If you should default on payments at some time in the future, the bank might have to sell the property to get its money. From your viewpoint, it would be better to get 75 or 80 percent or even more, if possible, to avoid an excessive outlay of your own funds.

The duration of the loan is the second important item to consider. It's usually to your advantage to obtain as long a term as possible. Since ours is an inflationary economy, the more time you have to pay off a loan, the cheaper will be the dollars with which you pay. If possible, aim for a payout period of 20 years or longer.

The banker, too, knows about inflation. He may want to keep the term of the loan relatively short for the same reason you want it long. He wants to be repaid before the value of the loan is greatly reduced by inflation.

The interest rate of the loan will depend partly on the current state of the money market, which determines the rate at which the banker must borrow the money to lend to you. It will also depend on supply and demand for loans in that community at that time. (Some lenders are now using *variable-rate* mortgages to protect themselves from widely fluctuating interest rates. Such mortgages are discussed later in this chapter.)

The use of *points* is another means by which the bank obtains additional income. In the example described above, the banker said that he would make a loan at "14 and three." This means that the interest rate is 14 percent, and in addition, you'll have to pay three points. A point is one percent of the face amount of the mortgage. If your mortgage is $350,000 (70 percent of $500,000), three points would be $10,500, to be paid at the time of the closing, when the mortgage is formally granted to you. Since you'll be receiving $350,000 but immediately paying back $10,500, you're actually receiving $339,500 but agreeing to repay $350,000, with interest calculated on the whole $350,000. Obviously, points are to be avoided if possible. Lenders charge points if loan money is generally scarce and if they feel that the market—that's you—will accept the extra charge. The net effect of paying points is the same as if you were paying a higher rate of interest on the loan. On a 15-year loan, each point you pay at the start is the approximate equivalent of an extra 0.1 percent of interest over the life of the loan. If you must pay points, try to have them labeled as a cost that will be deductible. Ask your accountant about it.

The final implication in the banker's reply is that the loan is contingent on your being an acceptable credit risk. You'll be asked to complete a detailed personal financial statement of your income, assets, outstanding debts, and net worth. Ordinarily, doctors are considered excellent credit risks, but if you or your partners are already deeply in debt, the bank may be concerned about your ability to repay another large loan.

NEGOTIATING A LOAN: STRATEGY AND TACTICS

The first step in obtaining financing for your building should be to call several banks in your area. The imaginary conversation presented above can serve as a guide. Once you have an idea of the terms available, you can plan your approach. Your strategy should be based on these facts:

1. The banker wants your other business besides this long-term loan: your business checking account, your savings account, your long-term certificates of deposit (possibly from your pension or Keogh plan), and your short-term auto and home-improvement loans. If you can show that you have been a regular customer for many years, this may help. Surprisingly, though, you can sometimes negotiate a better loan with a bank with which you have not previously done business. A new banker may look forward to obtaining all your other business, while your present banker may be taking you for granted. You should let a new banker know that if you receive favorable terms on this loan he can expect your other business. You might also let your present banker know that if he cannot offer you this loan on favorable terms, you might have to take your other business elsewhere.

2. The banker is concerned with the safety of his loan. The more you can prove to him that you are secure financially, the happier he will be to grant it on your terms.

3. The terms first quoted to you by the loan officer are not final. They are negotiable.

4. It's whom you know! This unfortunate fact of life applies to this situation. If you're well known to one or more members of the bank's board of directors or loan committee you'll have someone speaking on your behalf when your mortgage application is considered. It probably won't make the difference between the granting or refusal of your mortgage, but if a member of the loan committee can speak well of you and your prospects you may get your mortgage on more favorable terms.

With these points in mind, you can consider the following tactics:

1. Make a list of all your strong points. These should include your personal assets, your present income, and your projected future income; the amounts—in the form of Keogh or pension money—you're likely to be able to deposit in the bank now and in the future; your status in the community as a leader in civic, social, and/or religious organizations; and any other positive information about yourself and your project.

2. Concentrate on the banks that are likely to offer the best loan terms. These may well be the ones at which you have personal contacts. From each, ask for a loan application and a personal financial statement form.

3. When you submit the loan application and personal financial statement, send along your building plans and specifications and a covering letter. *This letter can be very important.* In it you should:

☐ include all the information you have noted about your present situation and future prospects on the list drawn up earlier;

☐ ask for a loan on terms *more favorable* to you than those quoted by the loan officer to whom you first spoke (if you were told the bank's terms were a 70 percent loan for 15 years at 14 percent and three points, request an 80 percent loan for 20 years at 11 percent with no points); and

☐ point out how the bank is likely to benefit by granting you the loan.

When the bank receives your formal application and letter, it will be discussed at a meeting of the appropriate group in the bank. Depending on the bank's size and its policy, this group will probably be the board of directors or the loan committee. Before the meeting, the loan officer will order a report about your credit standing from the local credit bureau. He'll also ask the bank's appraiser to review your plans and specifications and to provide him with an appraisal of the finished value of the building and land.

The response of the loan committee will depend on many factors, including your credit standing, your net worth, the length of time you've been in the community, the terms you are seeking, the state of the money market, and how much your business is likely to mean to the bank.

The committee's decision will be reported to you by the loan officer. It may be a firm No to your request for any kind of loan; it may be near-total acquiescence to your requests; depending on how much clout you have, it may be somewhere in between.

The committee's response may not be its final word. Don't be awed by its pronouncements. If you want some aspect of your project reviewed again, send another letter, asking the committee to reconsider its decision. Remember that the committee probably wants you as a customer, but its members are trying to get the best deal possible for the bank.

In your second letter, you might accept some of the bank's terms but still hold out against others. You might even make additional demands of your own. For example, you may agree to a higher interest rate than you originally requested and, at the same time, insist that the tax escrow account be waived. This is an account most banks demand of mortgagors. It consists of monthly payments in addition to the principal and interest of mortgage payments. The bank uses this escrow money to pay taxes on the property when due, but since taxes are paid only a few times each year, and the escrow money accumulates each month, the bank earns income with this money. In some states, little or no interest is paid on the escrow money to the mortgagor. It is far better for you to pay the taxes directly. In this way, you can earn income on the money as it accumulates before tax time. The banker may act appalled at such a request, but many banks waive these accounts for favored customers.

It's impossible to describe all the variations possible in these negotiations. Unless you're certain that one particular lender is offering you the best possible terms, you should shop at two or three banks for your loan. Local pension funds and insurance companies are other possible sources. It may surprise you how much their terms vary from one another.

Finally, you must be aware of several other points:

1. The amount of the loan will be based on a real-estate appraiser's estimate of the *market value* of the completed project, *not on what you will pay for it.* His appraisal will be based on, among other things, the size, location, and likely demand for your building and on the materials to be used. He will neither know nor care how high the bids run when builders review your plans and specifications. If he appraises your project at $450,000 and you have a 70 percent commitment from the bank, it will lend you $315,000. Even if the lowest construction bid plus the cost of the land total $500,000, the bank is not likely to increase the amount of your mortgage. This is why you need an architect who knows both current construction costs and the market values of professional buildings. The closer your costs come to the appraiser's estimate, the less out-of-pocket expenses you'll have.

2. When your loan is approved, it'll be called a *construction loan* during the time your building is going up. When it's completed and you've moved in, it'll be converted to a conventional mortgage. During construction, you'll be asked to pay accrued interest each quarter on the amount of the loan that has been advanced to you.

The loan arrangements I've described in this chapter are those that occur when the same lender provides the money for construction and for a long-term mortgage. This is customary in some suburban and rural areas. In many cities, though, you'll get only your construction loan at a bank. The interest rate will be pegged to the prime rate—one or two points above it. The long-term mortgage will have to be found elsewhere, usually with the help of a mortgage broker. He'll find a lender for your project among the insurance companies or pension funds with which he has contacts. Naturally, you'll pay a commission for this service.

3. The construction loan won't be turned over to you as a lump sum. Rather, it'll be doled out as construction continues. The process often works something like this: The builder submits a requisition for payment to your architect. The architect inspects the job to see that the claimed amount of work has been done. When he approves a payment, you ask the bank for a portion of your loan. The bank now sends its appraiser to evaluate the completed work. Once again, the appraiser is interested only in protecting the bank's investment. He'll estimate what percent of the work is completed and what percent remains to be done. He may also estimate how much money would be needed in reserve to complete the project if the builder suddenly walked off the job or went bankrupt. Based on these figures, he'll recommend that the bank advance to you a specific dollar amount or a specific percent of the total loan. After the title company reassures the bank that you're still the owner of the property, the bank will advance the money to you. Any difference between this amount and the amount owed to the builder must come from you.

4. At the formal granting of the construction loan (or later, when it's converted to a mortgage), you'll be asked to pay certain amounts to the bank. These may include survey charges, appraiser's fees, bank legal fees, mortgage taxes, title insurance, and other costs. Be prepared!

5. The type of mortgage discussed thus far is known as a *fixed-rate, self-amortizing* mortgage. *Fixed-rate* means that the interest rate will stay constant throughout the term of the mortgage. *Self-amortizing* means that the monthly payments are such that at the end of the term the loan will be paid off.

There are other types of mortgages, two of which are worth mentioning. A *variable-rate* or *rollover* mortgage is one in which the interest rate may change at specified intervals. It became popular with lenders in 1979-80, when interest rates zoomed upward.

Try to get a fixed-rate mortgage, if such a mortgage is still available. You may have to take a rollover type if banks phase out fixed-rate mortgages.

A *balloon* mortgage is one you might want to try for. Instead of paying off the mortgage in equal monthly installments, you pay a smaller amount each month and a lump sum—the balloon—at the end. The advantage of this type of loan is that you put inflation to work for you. The lump sum will be paid in dollars that are worth less than dollars are now. Of course, when it comes due, you may want to refinance that balloon for an additional period.

One way to arrange for a balloon, if you are offered a 15-year mortgage, is to ask for a 15-year term with a 20-year payout. The monthly payments would be those of a 20-year self-amortizing mortgage, but since you pay them for only 15 years, there will be a balloon left at the end.

6. A requirement that you should try to avoid is the *construction holdback*. A lender may insist on withholding part of the construction loan until you can show that a certain percentage—say 80 percent—of the building has been leased. This presents no problem if all offices will be occupied by owner-tenants. But if you build extra space, it'll mean that you'll have to find those other tenants promptly or find some extra cash until you do.

7. Even if the entity putting up your building is a corporation or a partnership, you and each of the other owners will almost certainly be required by the lender to guarantee the loan personally.

8. Some lenders insist on receiving a share of the building's equity or profits as a sweetener for granting the loan. This is a method the lenders use to cope with inflation. Try to keep it out of the mortgage contract.

9. In your negotiations, try to avoid a *prepayment penalty* or try to keep it low. If your building must be sold before the mortgage is paid off, you'll want the right to prepay the outstanding balance with as little penalty as possible. Similarly, if you wish to refinance the building at a later date, you'll want to repay the existing mortgage.

IV
PRELIMINARY PLANS

19
YOUR OFFICE: WISH LISTS AND CHECKLISTS

Throughout the rest of the book, I've kept the discussion of the planning, design, and construction of the *office* separate from the discussion of the *building*. The planning of your office has to be essentially the same, whether you rent, renovate, or build from the ground up, and if you erect a new building you have to plan, design, and construct it and your office simultaneously. But I've separated the two so you can skip the parts that don't apply to you.

I use the word architect here to designate the person in charge of the planning and design. If you use the services of a space planner, an interior architect, or a supply-house planning department (as discussed in Chapter 3) instead of a registered A.I.A. architect, just mentally insert the title of your expert where you read architect.

The best way to begin the planning process is to write a *wish list*, a compilation of everything you might possibly want—within reason—in your new office. Later, you'll separate the "must" items from those that depend on cost.

There's another reason for starting with a wish list. It'll clarify your thoughts about what you really want. The more detailed it is, the better, for it'll give the architect a more accurate concept of what you're after. It reduces the likelihood of overlooking something in the early planning stages that might be difficult to add later.

Take the list with you to the planning sessions with the architect. It can serve as the starting point for your discussion. Save it to review later on, to see if all the points on it have been covered.

As you bring up each item on your list, the architect will—or should—question you about it.

"How do you know you need a waiting room seating 10 patients?

"How long are your appointments? Do you keep on schedule? How far behind do you get? How many people, on the average, accompany each patient into the waiting room?

"What is a comfortable size for a treatment room? What will you put in it? How big is the equipment? Is it fixed or movable? How many people are likely to be in a treatment room at one time?"

The architect's questions will sharpen your own thinking about what you want and need. Your answers will give him the beginnings of his *program*. Architects speak in terms of *programs*, *problems*, and *solutions*. The program in this case is the number and size of the rooms, their functions, and how they relate to each other. The problem is to fit them together in the best way. His solutions are the floor plans and other drawings he prepares for you and, with your help, revises until your needs are satisfied.

By the end of your first or second meeting, you and the architect will have agreed on how large an office—in square feet—you should have. To arrive at this figure he adds together all the desirable room sizes and then adds an additional percentage to accommodate partitions, hallways, and similar space. This is essentially what we did in Table 1-1, but now your needs should be more clearly defined.

Before the architect can begin to develop a floor plan or plans, both of you have to focus on the concepts of *zones* and *traffic patterns* in your office.

A zone is a part of the office devoted to a specific major function. Each zone should be situated so the operations to which it is dedicated can be done efficiently and without interference from—or interfering with—the performance of functions in other zones.

Traffic patterns refer to the movements within and between zones. A good traffic pattern exists when people (patients, doctors, and staff) can safely reach destinations in the office with maximum efficiency for office procedures, without bumping into one another, and with proper consideration for one another's sensitivities.

Figures 19-1 to 19-4 show how our office floor plan developed from zones. Note these points on the final floor plan:

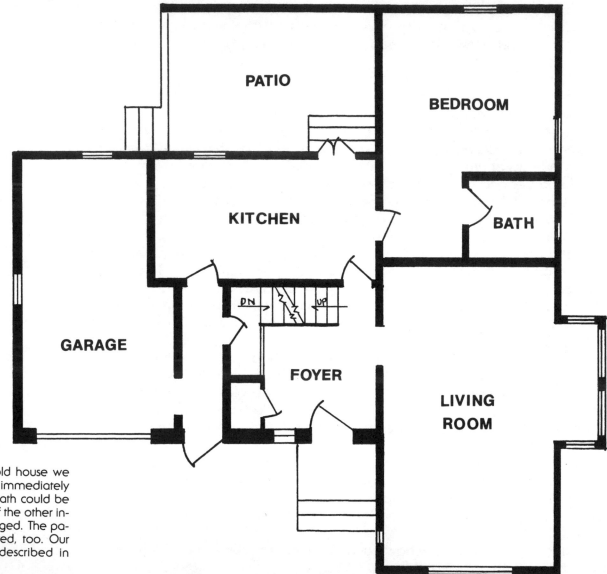

Figure 19-1. Floor plan, first floor of old house we bought in 1976. We suspected almost immediately that the living room, bedroom, and bath could be left more or less intact, but that most of the other interior partitions would have to be changed. The patio would probably have to be removed, too. Our experience with the construction is described in Chapter 62.

☐ The reception room and the patients' lavatory are separate from the rest of the office.

☐ The business office is the buffer between the reception room and the remainder of the office. It's placed so that all patients must pass it when entering and leaving.

☐ The treatment zone is an L-shaped group of rooms on the north and east sides of the office, away from both reception area and business office.

☐ The two doctors share a private office, which is situated between two pairs of treatment rooms.

☐ Two treatment rooms used by hygienists are accessible by a separate hallway from the waiting room.

☐ Support services—central supply/sterilization/darkroom—are centrally located and easily accessible to assistants moving through the treatment zone.

☐ The staff lounge and staff lavatory are separate from the rest of the office.

We find that this zone arrangement works well for us. It isn't necessarily the best plan possible, but it permits our office functions to be carried out comfortably, efficiently, and with few unnecessary steps.

Your traffic flow and your zones may be quite unlike ours. Different specialties have different needs. My reason for showing you ours is to emphasize that as you and your architect begin your preliminary planning, you should think first in terms of zones rather than individual rooms. Think about how these zones should relate to one another and how a patient or doctor or staff member will travel within the zones and between them.

Your architect knows that in order for your traffic pattern to be comfortable and efficient you'll need:

☐ adequate room size;

☐ adequate width of doorways and halls;

☐ adequate space between and around pieces of furniture and equipment;

☐ collision-free corners and no people-stoppers, such as bulletin boards and cosmetic mirrors, in the traffic stream;

☐ the receptionist's desk in a location where entering patients can easily announce their arrival and where departing patients can make future appointments and payments;

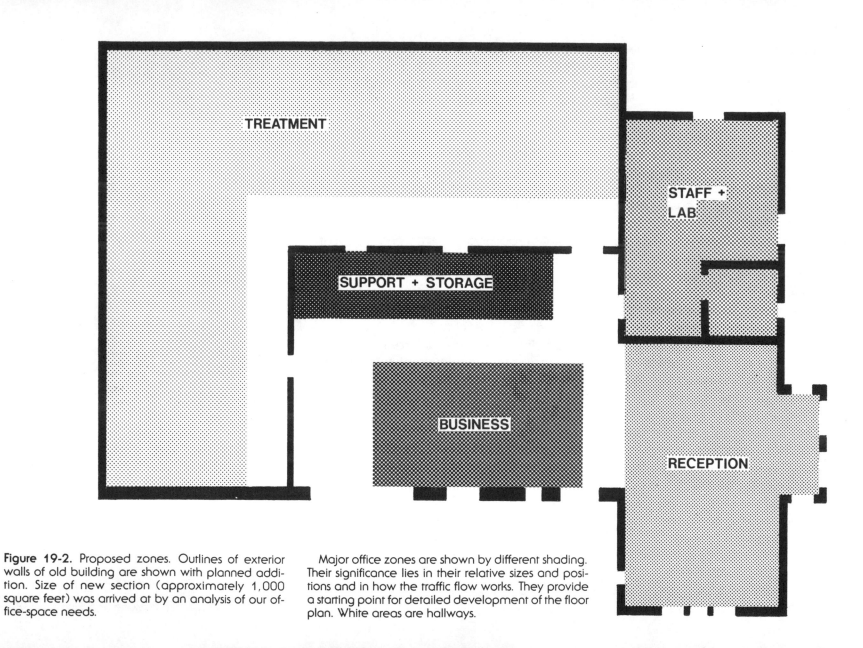

TREATMENT

STAFF + LAB

SUPPORT + STORAGE

BUSINESS

RECEPTION

Figure 19-2. Proposed zones. Outlines of exterior walls of old building are shown with planned addition. Size of new section (approximately 1,000 square feet) was arrived at by an analysis of our office-space needs.

Major office zones are shown by different shading. Their significance lies in their relative sizes and positions and in how the traffic flow works. They provide a starting point for detailed development of the floor plan. White areas are hallways.

☐ extra floor space in areas where people are likely to congregate, such as in front of a receptionist's desk, to avoid bottlenecks and crowding;

☐ no doors opening into the traffic stream;

☐ equipment and doorways placed to protect patients' privacy; and

☐ "emotional" space—a little extra space in a room, a hall, or a vestibule beyond what is merely adequate.

In addition, traffic flow may be improved by keeping patient and staff traffic patterns separate from each other whenever possible.

Architectural drawings include several views:

☐ a *plan*—a bird's-eye view looking down on the office or the building;

☐ an *elevation*—a view of a vertical facade such as a wall, either interior or exterior;

☐ a *section*—a cutaway view of a structure, showing the vertical and horizontal relationship of parts; and

☐ a *perspective*—an attempt to show how a building or room will look in three dimensions.

When you receive the first drawings, review them carefully. Do they show *all* the zones? Do the zones appear to be properly sized? Keep a ruler or architect's scale handy to translate the drawings into full-sized dimensions so you can visualize what they will look like. Are the zones in the proper relationship to each other? Does the traffic flow appear correct?

On the plan that seems best, make whatever changes you think are required. Don't be afraid to reject all of the sketches if the architect seems not to have caught the spirit of what you're after; but don't dismiss a design only because it's different from anything you have previously seen or considered. These early sketches give you something specific to discuss with the architect. Later drawings will become progressively more detailed.

If you are erecting a single office building, keep in mind the future resale of the building. Oddly shaped or oddly sized rooms will make the building harder to sell.

If your office will be in your own multioffice building, remember that you may need more space in the future. You can sometimes prepare for this by renting the office next to yours to a nonowner. By establishing lease lengths

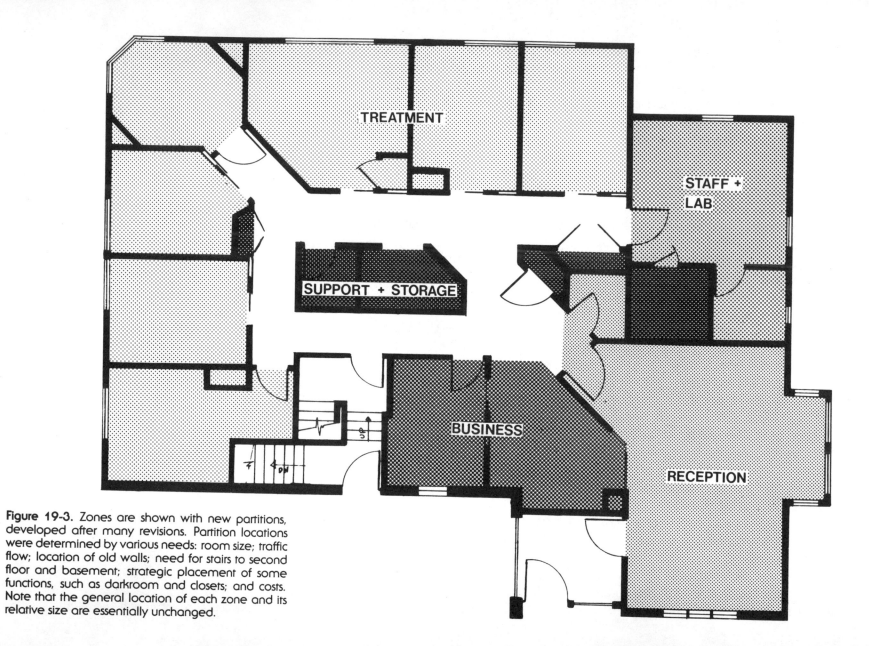

Figure 19-3. Zones are shown with new partitions, developed after many revisions. Partition locations were determined by various needs: room size; traffic flow; location of old walls; need for stairs to second floor and basement; strategic placement of some functions, such as darkroom and closets; and costs. Note that the general location of each zone and its relative size are essentially unchanged.

with your needs in mind, you can arrange for the space to be available if and when you need it.

On the pages that follow are *wish-list* and *checklist* questions and ideas for each major part of your office. Use the first group to give you ideas for preparing your own wish list about each area. By doing your homework in this way you'll probably reduce the number and length of preliminary meetings with the architect.

Use the checklist questions when you review the drawings prepared by the architect. They'll keep you from overlooking some important item.

As you think about each part of the office, try to envision what's ahead for your practice five to 10 years down the road. Are you likely to take on an additional associate or more? Will you need more office help for the deluge of insurance claims, tax forms, and other assorted paperwork that is virtually certain to increase? Will the expanded use of assistants make more exam/treatment rooms desirable? Plan ahead, but don't go overboard.

Most of the items in the following lists are appropriate for either a medical or a dental office. A few are pertinent only for one or the other. For some additional details to consider, see Chapters 37 and 57.

RECEPTION-ROOM WISH LIST

How many seats are needed? If you often are behind schedule you need extra seats. If patients are often accompanied to your office by others, those friends or relatives must also be seated. Take into account possible future changes in routines and addition of associates.

How large a coat rack will you need? Usually, there should be one coat-hanging space for each chair in the waiting room.

Will you want tables or racks for reading matter?

Do you have any special lighting needs? For example, older people need more light for reading comfortably.

Do you want a children's alcove with small-scale furniture? This is probably a must in the office of a pediatrician or a pedodontist. Other practices will also find such an area useful.

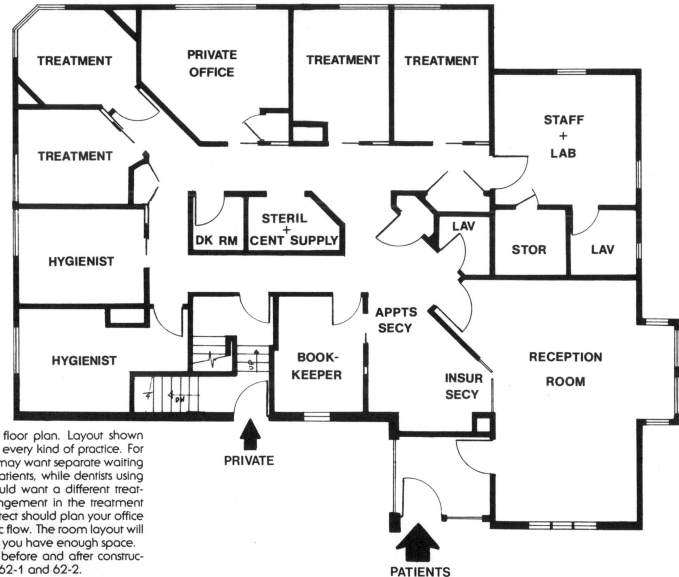

Figure 19-4. Final office floor plan. Layout shown would not be suitable for every kind of practice. For example, a pediatrician may want separate waiting rooms for sick and well patients, while dentists using the T.E.A.M. concept would want a different treatment room/corridor arrangement in the treatment zone. You and your architect should plan your office based on zones and traffic flow. The room layout will then develop naturally, if you have enough space.

Photos of our building before and after construction are shown in Figures 62-1 and 62-2.

Will you need an area for patients to fill out insurance forms?
Is a signal system needed to indicate the arrival and departure of patients?

RECEPTION-ROOM CHECKLIST

Is the room large enough to seat the patient load expected? Generally, architects use about 15 to 20 square feet per person for estimating reception-
room size. This provides for seating plus tables and other furniture as well as
clear space for leg room and walking. However, the number of square feet
is often less important than the shape of the room and the amount of avail-
able wall space.
Is the room apart from the rest of the office? It should be.
Does it have one or more windows facing outside? A pleasing view is nice to
have, but not always possible.
Is the patients' lavatory close to the reception room?
Is the room planned to allow for clusters of seating rather than rows of chairs?
Is there a children's alcove?
Is the doorway wide enough to admit a wheelchair?
Is there a separate private entrance in addition to the one that opens into the
reception room?
If patients are to enter the office directly from outdoors Is there a vestibule or
lobby to prevent drafts?
Is there a need for separate areas for sick and well patients?
Has the patients' coat area been identified?
Are all parts of the room visible from the business office?

BUSINESS-OFFICE WISH LIST

How many people will work here?
What kinds of work will they do?
    Schedule appointments on phone?
    Schedule appointments in person?
    Receive payments?
    Record payments?

File and retrieve patients' records?
Handle insurance claims?
Type?
Bookkeeping?
Photocopying?
What furniture and equipment will be needed?
  Desks? Chairs? How many?
  File cabinets?
    Type: vertical or lateral? If lateral,
      fixed-shelf or drawer type?
    Size: letter? legal?
  Is a work surface needed for assembling groups
    of charts?
  Typewriters?
    Size?
    Number?
  Dictating equipment?
  Telephones?
  Answering machine?
  Photocopier?
  Postage meter? Postage scale?
  Computer terminal(s)?
  Special lighting needs?

BUSINESS-OFFICE CHECKLIST

Is it large enough? Providing inadequate space here is one of the most frequent
  failures in professional-office planning. According to management consultants, the rule of thumb here is to provide 100 square feet for a one-secretary
  office and about 75 square feet more for each additional person who will
  work here. The final figure depends partly on how much equipment is to be
  in the area now and in the future.
will the receptionist at her desk have a clear view of the entry door, the waiting
  room, and the patients' coat rack?

Will she have enough privacy so that her phone conversations are not overheard by those in the waiting room?

Will arriving and departing patients have to pass her desk to announce their arrival, to make future appointments, and to make payments?

Will she be able to reach the most actively used patient records without leaving her desk or with only a few steps?

Will she be able to discuss financial matters with a patient without being overheard by patients in the waiting room?

Will she be in a position to be aware of the doctor's progress so she can monitor patient flow?

If the office is to have a bookkeeper and/or a business manager, does that person have a space that can be closed off for privacy and for discussing accounts with patients?

If two or more assistants are to work in this area, will each have her own defined area? (See Chapter 45.)

Can patient records be pulled from the files by anyone in this area?

PRIVATE-OFFICE/CONSULTATION-ROOM WISH LIST

How large do you want it?

What will be in it?

Desk? (how large?)

Chairs? (how many?)

Recliner easy chair?

File cabinets?

X-ray view box?

Bookshelves?

Corkboard?

Chalkboard?

What will you use it for?

Patient consultations?

Private business?

Study?

Relaxation?

Private lavatory needed? Shower?
Special lighting?
Special audiovisual needs for patient education?
Soundproofing?
If there are or will be two or more doctors, will you need a separate private office for each doctor or one common office? Usually this depends on what you intend to use it for and whether both doctors will be working at the same time.

PRIVATE-OFFICE/CONSULTATION-ROOM CHECKLIST

Is it large enough for what you plan to have in it now and in the future?
Is it situated close to the treatment rooms to minimize walking?
Is it situated away from the waiting room for privacy?
Does it contain a coat closet for your use?

EXAM/TREATMENT-ROOMS WISH LIST

How many are needed now and will be needed in the future?
What is optimum size?
Is it necessary to have a window in each?
What equipment must be in each one? List all items with approximate sizes, including mobile equipment such as operating stools and instrument carts.
Should there be a special dressing area? The spaciousness and comfort of this area is important in OB/GYN practices.
Built-ins?
Special plumbing?
Special electrical needs?
Special lighting?

EXAM/TREATMENT-ROOMS CHECKLIST

Are they located away from the waiting room? Are they close to your private office? Will you have enough of them?
Is the room size correct? You will want enough area for all of the equipment and built-ins required, with sufficient space to move in, out, and around the

room. Avoid excess space that only lessens efficiency. Sizes frequently range between 80 and 120 square feet, but may vary in some specialties. Don't be afraid to consider imaginative shapes if they will increase efficiency and avoid wasted space.

To assure that the room size you select will be correct for your equipment, measure any equipment you now have or new equipment you are likely to buy and draw its outlines to scale on one-quarter-inch graph paper. If you cut out these outlines and reinforce them with cardboard or oaktag glued to the back you'll be able to shift them around into different arrangements on your floor plan.

Will your proposed placement of equipment permit efficient traffic flow within the room? If you'll have to push a piece of equipment into a cabinet and close the door each time a patient enters or leaves the room, your room or your equipment or both are poorly designed.

The following dimensions may be useful in your planning:

☐ walking space, if needed, between pieces of cabinetry or equipment: 30 inches or more;

☐ minimum space for an assistant to work on the side of patient opposite doctor: 30 to 36 inches;

☐ usual countertop depth, front-to-back: 18 inches.

Are all treatment rooms approximately the same size and shape? For maximum efficiency, you should want identical or similar pieces of equipment placed in the same location in each room.

Are the doorways placed with proper attention to your patients' need for privacy? If your patients must undress, has a dressing area been provided that can be curtained or otherwise screened off? If treatment rooms are on either side of a hallway, soundproofing will be improved if the doors are not directly opposite each other.

If you have a dental practice that uses the T.E.A.M. (Training in Expanded Auxiliary Management) approach, has the treatment area been planned for maximum efficiency? More information on this subject can be found in books on the T.E.A.M. concept.

Don't get hung up on the notion that the best way to design neighboring treatment rooms or lavatories is with sinks back-to-back. While you can save a bit on plumbing with this approach, it's false economy if you do it with little regard for convenience and traffic flow. The plumbing expense is a one-time cost, while a badly placed fixture will annoy you every time you use it.

LABORATORY WISH LIST

What procedures will be done here?
What equipment will be needed? List them.
How many people will work here at one time?
Will there be more than one full-time technician?
Will the workers be sitting or standing?
What room or rooms should be close to or next to the lab?
Will the room serve any other function, such as darkroom, staff lounge, central supply area, sterilization?
Special lighting?
Special plumbing?
Special electrical needs?
Special floor covering?
Soundproofing needed?
Odor control needed?
Dust control needed?

LABORATORY CHECKLIST

Is the room large enough to serve all intended functions? Is it located properly for good traffic flow?

LAVATORIES WISH LIST

How many are needed?
  Patients?
  Staff?
  Doctor(s)?

Any special facilities needed?

In a medical office where urine specimens are needed, a convenient location for the patients' lavatory is sometimes next to the lab. A pass-through in the shared wall with a small door on each side permits delivery of the specimen without the need for carrying it through the hall.

LAVATORIES CHECKLIST

Does patients' lavatory have a door wide enough for a wheelchair?
Is there enough floor space for a wheelchair inside?
Is the location appropriate?
Is staff lavatory close to staff lounge?

DARKROOM WISH LIST

Do you need one? If you use daylight-loading automatic processors, you may think you don't need a darkroom. My own view is that a darkroom—with tanks—is desirable as a backup to the processor. It's still essential at present for duplicating dental films to be sent to insurance companies.

The darkroom should be close to the rooms that have X-ray machines.

How large a room? It should be at least big enough for two people to stand side by side at the work surface with door closed. This permits an assistant to teach darkroom procedures to a new employee. Five feet by five feet is probably adequate.

Are there special electrical needs?

Do you need special plumbing? A water mixing valve?

DARKROOM CHECKLIST

Is the size correct? Is the location correct?

STORAGE-SPACE WISH LIST

You can never have too much storage space, but you'll regret not having enough. Most doctors don't allow sufficient space for storage in new offices because they underestimate their needs. Below is a list of the sort of things you'll need either to store or at least place temporarily in closets or cabinets. Some of the categories overlap.

How much space will you need for storing:

Patient records: Active and inactive? How much additional file space is needed each year? How often are the records culled?

Business, insurance, and tax records, current and noncurrent?

Blank stationery, insurance, business and patient record forms?

Office supplies?

Disposable paper and plastic supplies?

Instruments?

Medications?

Clinical photographic equipment and supplies?

Emergency supplies?

Daily supplies for patient care, including tray set-ups?

Laboratory supplies?

Tools, spare parts for equipment?

Office cleaning equipment, supplies?

Staff clothing, uniforms?

Doctors' clothing, uniforms?

Trash not yet removed from office?

Other items?

Will any storage areas have to be kept locked?

You'll have to work out your own space needs for each of these groups, but we've found that these storage ideas work for us:

1. Our most valuable storage space isn't in the office proper but in the basement of our building's new wing.

This 1,000 square foot, dry, heated space is accessible from the office by a flight of stairs. It has a separate outside entrance just a few steps below ground level. The separate entrance permits deliveries of bulky items without going through the office.

Here we keep records of patients who have died, left the practice, or are seen very infrequently as well as old business and tax records. Inexpensive steel shelves are used to hold paper and plastic disposables, stationery, and other supplies. The space permits us to order in large quantities and to take advantage of discounts. We don't come close to needing all the space right now for office purposes, so it's a great place to store rarely used bulky items from our home basements. It's also worthwhile, and relatively inexpensive, to have a file-storage room built in your basement to protect your inactive records from dust and fire.

The point is to have a dry, heated storage area that is outside the office, yet easily accessible. If no such place is available, you'll need more storage room in the office, possibly much more, depending on the type and size of your practice. My guess is that you'll need about 10 percent of your total office area for storage, *not* including the floor space taken by file cabinets, desks, and built-in cabinets in your treatment rooms.

2. A policy of regularly culling our active-patient-record file cabinets prevents them from becoming overloaded. We find that about 80 folders occupy 12 linear inches of shelf space. Thus, for every 80 charts pulled from the files, we need another foot of inactive file storage. Also, we need one to two linear feet of file drawer space each year for the business, payroll tax, and pension records and ledgers. Those likely to be needed are kept in the office, while the older ones are stored in the basement in the cartons (12" × 24" × 12" high) that we used for moving.

3. We store supplies, enough for at least several days or a few weeks, as close as possible to where they are used. Business-office supplies and stationery are in metal two-shelf *overfile* cabinets with sliding doors. These rest on top of our five-drawer lateral file cabinets (see Figure 41-3). Copying supplies are kept in a smaller cabinet under our photocopy machine. Central supply (see Figure 42-3 3B), which is also the sterilization area, is the source from which the assistants fill the cabinets in each treatment room. The darkroom has its own supply shelves. A centrally located closet provides space for gas tanks and emergency supplies. Two other small closets are used for staff coats and uniforms and doctors' coats. A large walk-in closet with shelves on three sides contains backup supplies, seldom-used items, spare parts and tools for quick repairs, as well as cleaning equipment and supplies.

4. Trash storage (see Chapter 27) is a problem for us, since our village picks up garbage only once a week. We keep the volume down by using a trash compactor.

STORAGE-SPACE CHECKLIST

Has the architect provided ample space for storage of each of the items mentioned earlier in the wish list? Go through the list and check it against the plans.

Will you have adequate aisle space for each storage area? In a walk-in closet, for example, you need at least a two-foot-wide aisle to permit access to the rear of the closet. Where file cabinets are used, a minimum two-foot space for the user is needed in front of the file. If the file drawers or shelves pull out, you need more aisle space in front of them, and if other staff members walk through this area, additional space is needed to prevent collisions.

Is the space allotted to each kind of item appropriate for it? You probably won't want to put many different small items, such as drug samples, on a few deep shelves. More but shallower shelves may be better. Since your needs may change, specify adjustable shelves.

Have you calculated your file cabinet needs in terms of the number of linear feet of file drawer space needed for active records? for inactive records? Has the appropriate floor space been provided?

Are you planning to rely heavily on storage in built-in cabinet drawers for treatment-room items? Think twice: Built-in or mobile cabinets covered with plastic laminate are soaring in price. Keep your cabinet needs down to the essentials and consider using tray set-ups from a large central supply area.

HALLWAYS WISH LIST

Be sure your halls are wide enough. Five-foot width is best. Three and one-half feet is too narrow for anything but a short hallway. No matter how large your rooms are, your office will feel cramped if the halls are too narrow. Narrow halls make collisions much more likely. You won't regret a little extra "emotional" space.

HALLWAYS CHECKLIST

Are the halls wide enough? Are they at their widest where people may congregate, such as at the receptionist's desk?
Are they arranged to avoid collisions?

UTILITY-ROOM WISH LIST

What will the room contain?
  Heating, ventilating, and air-conditioning equipment?
  Janitor's sink?
  Hot-water heater?
  Central suction?
  Air compressor?
  Storage?
How much space will be needed? You and your architect may not be able to decide this until your mechanical needs are fully analyzed.
Soundproofing needed? Since this room is likely to have noise-producing equipment, it should be as far away as possible from patient-care areas.

UTILITY-ROOM CHECKLIST

Is size adequate? Is location suitable?
Have local regulations been checked to find out if there are limitations to placement of this equipment?
Will special fire protection be needed in walls and door?

SPECIAL-ROOMS WISH LIST

Will you need any of these special rooms? Try to combine functions wherever possible.
Bookkeeper's office?
Office manager's office?
Recovery room(s)?
  How many?
  Size?

Location?
What equipment, furniture needed?
Sterilization area?
  How much room needed?
  Equipment needed?
    Sink?
    Ultrasonic cleaner?
    Sterilizer? Size?
  How much counter space needed?
  Place so soiled or bloody instruments are not seen by passing patients.
Audiovisual room for patient education?
Staff lounge?
  Separate room or part of another?
  Furniture and equipment?
    Table and chairs?
    Refrigerator?
    Sink?
    Hot plate?
    Coffee maker?
Special medical office areas?
  Nurses' station?
  Cast room?
  EEG?
  X-ray?
  Minor surgery?
  Other?
Special dental office areas?
  Panographic X-ray alcove?
  Hygienist room(s)?
  Preventive therapist room?
  For each special area, list name of room, ideal size, number of people normally using it, furniture and equipment needed, most desirable location in relation to other areas, special plumbing, electrical, and lighting needs.

20
YOUR BUILDING: WISH LIST AND CHECKLIST

Your needs and desires concerning the building will probably be vague compared to those relating to your own office, but it will still be helpful to the architect if you and your partners, if you have any, express your feelings about the points covered in this chapter.

WISH LIST

Size. The maximum building size may be already determined by the size of the lot and the local zoning code, but if yours is a large piece of property you may want to consider a modest-size building now with the option of an addition later.

Buildings can be enlarged either horizontally or vertically. If you hope to expand vertically in the future, your original structure needs a stronger foundation, a more rigid framework, and unused elevator shafts, all of which cost more money. Moreover, this extra capacity may never be used.

Horizontal expansion doesn't entail structural preparations, but it requires a larger initial outlay for extra land. This additional land must be enough for building a new wing plus increased parking space. If you decide later that you won't enlarge your building, you can probably sell the extra property.

Style. Do you have any inclinations for contemporary, colonial, Spanish, or other style of architecture?

Exterior material. Is there any particular material that you prefer? Brick? Stone? Wood? Aluminum siding?

Special features. Have you always wanted a skylight? An atrium for plants? Some other special construction? Now is the time to say so.

Storage. Try to get as much unfinished storage space as possible. Read the section on storage in the previous chapter. If yours is a multioffice building, available storage space will make it more attractive to prospective tenants. Consider dividing the open basement or other storage area into partitioned bins or rooms that can be locked by the user. Be sure the architect knows that the area must be dry and kept at a comfortable temperature.

THE NEEDS OF THE HANDICAPPED

Federal, state, and local laws now require what is known as "barrier-free construction." This means that any physical barriers that might prevent the use of a building by a handicapped person are prohibited. The following passage was originally printed in the *Journal of the American Dental Association*, March 1979. Copyright by the American Dental Association. Reprinted by permission. This abbreviated version of federal regulations applies to all office buildings. In some localities, the requirements are stricter. Your architect should be able to provide more detailed information.

"The federal government has set minimum standards for accessibility for physically disabled persons. The following recommendations are consistent with these standards. . . .

"LOCATION. An office may present a barrier if it is located on a steep hill or if the access is by many steps.

"Parking should be nearby with special spaces reserved for the disabled. Parking lots should be arranged so that persons in wheelchairs can move directly to the entrance without having to wheel behind parked cars.

"For a person on crutches, or using a walking frame or in a wheelchair, the walkway should not have high, smooth, underturned, untextured curbs, nor should there be decorative, widely spaced flagstones. For ground floor entrance, there should be a ramp with a grade of no more than 5° if there is no handrail.

"ENTRANCE. All steps should be contrasted with red or orange to aid depth perception. A ramp's gradient must not rise more than one inch for every foot or 8°. A ramp needs a handrail and must be at least four feet wide to accom-

modate wheelchairs. Ramps should have nonslip surfaces and level spaces every 25 to 30 feet. Large expanses of concrete should be patterned to reduce glare.

"The entrance should be well lit to aid visual accommodation, and the doorway threshold should not exceed a height of a half inch. Loose or thick doormats are dangerous for older or disabled patients. Doors should open easily with a push or pull and should not be pressurized above six pounds of pressure. Double and revolving doors are difficult to operate.

"Hallways should be well lit, with no low objects in the shadows. Elderly people need increased intensity of light, which must be without glare, in order to avoid accidents.

"A standard wheelchair is 42 inches long and 25 inches wide; the height of handles from the floor is 36 inches and the height of the seat from the floor is 20 inches. For a 360° turn, a wheelchair needs 54 inches. The average reach of an adult in a wheelchair is 60 inches vertically, 30 inches horizontally, and 48 inches diagonally from the floor. Therefore, for wheelchair maneuverability, a hallway must be at least five feet wide to allow for normal two-way traffic [of wheelchairs].

"*DIRECTORY AND PUBLIC PHONES.* The directory should be at eye level, positioned away from the glare of sunlight, with lettering of adequate size for easy readability. Phone dials and handles should be low, and booths should be accessible to a person in a wheelchair.

"*ELEVATORS.* To accommodate wheelchairs, elevators should be at least five by five feet with electric eyes that give people adequate time to enter and exit. The controls should be within the reach of a person in a wheelchair.

"*TOILETS AND WATER FOUNTAINS.* Toilet doors should swing outward, and safety handrails should be able to support at least 250 pounds.

"The toilet should be the height of a wheelchair, and the sink should be hung from the wall and be less than 34 inches high. For safety, the water temperature in the pipes should not exceed 120° F. Lever-type faucet handles are the easiest to operate. Water fountains should be operated by hand with controls in front. Recessed and alcove coolers are not recommended.

"*WAITING ROOM.* This area should be well lit without glare, and floors and walls should have contrasting colors. The floors should be level, with nonskid surfaces without deep carpets. There should not be low furniture or loose rugs, and chairs must not be soft or deep because disabled persons may not be able to get out of them."

CHECKLIST

The first drawings delivered by your architect will be rough sketches of plans that provide the square-foot area required and show how the building can be placed on the site. This is the first *site plan*. It will show the general arrangement for driveways and parking.

The architect may also provide some elevation or perspective drawings showing various types of exteriors, and your first interest will probably be in these drawings. At this stage, however, the site plan is more important.

Is the building size correct?

Has the architect chosen the best location for the building on the site? If it doesn't seem right, now is the time to question it. If necessary, go to the site with the architect to discuss it.

Has he taken advantage of a dramatic view? Does the position of the front entry make sense in relation to the street? To the parking area? Think about traffic flow outside the building.

On the first plans, the architect will probably block out the arrangement of the office suites and their relation to the lobby area. Do they all appear equally desirable from the standpoint of access? From the standpoint of view? If there are first-class and second-class suites, you may have problems with your partners over who gets which office.

Have the proper storage areas been provided?

Have the needs of the handicapped been provided for?

Once you've settled on the building's orientation and the general arrangement of suites, you can focus your attention on its outward appearance. This will be determined partly by your wishes and partly by costs.

From here on, the drawings will become more detailed as your conferences with the architect lead to refinements in the plan and elevations, to inclusion of mechanical needs, and to analysis and design of office suites.

21

CEILINGS AND FLOORS, WALLS AND DOORS

As the plans increase in detail, the architect will ask you for your preferences concerning the interior surfaces: walls, doors, ceilings, and floors. If you're erecting a building, you'll have to make decisions on many more items, but even in a rented suite you'll have to give some thought to the materials to be used. In this chapter, you'll learn of some of the choices you have. More details are presented in later chapters.

WALLS

Interior walls in your office will probably be built by erecting either vertical two-by-four wood studs or, where the fire code requires it, metal uprights that serve the same purpose. Over these, gypsum wallboard (often known by the trade name Sheetrock) is attached. The wallboard usually comes in four-by-12-foot panels that are one-half of an inch thick. It's produced by sandwiching a gypsum material between inner and outer paper layers. The joints where panels meet are covered by a special paper tape. Then the joints and the nails, which were hammered in slightly below the level of the outer surface of the wallboard, are covered with joint compound called spackle. The result is a smooth surface that can be painted, papered, or covered with plastic wallcovering. This type of partition is sometimes called *drywall* construction.

There are some variations in this method of wall construction that are used when maximum soundproofing is needed. These methods are discussed in Chapter 27.

Other materials can be used for interior walls, such as masonry block covered with plaster, or plastic panels. The initial cost, the installation difficulty, or the maintenance problems usually govern their use. One or another may be favored in some parts of the country.

Prefinished wood panels are easy to install, but you'd better stick to the better grades only. These usually have a tough finish that can be maintained with little effort.

If you've thought about some exotically shaped curved walls for parts of your office, find out the cost before giving the go-ahead. Most building materials are rectangular and are easiest to use for rectangular, flat surfaces. If a rounded wall is desired, considerable time and labor will be needed to convert the wallboard or paneling or other rectangular material to the curved form. Costs can jump astronomically.

Another consideration, if this is your own new building, is that strangely shaped walls and rooms could make your building harder to sell when that time comes.

Your principal concern about partitions should be that they look good, that they can be maintained easily, and, if acoustics are a concern, that they block sound transmission.

CEILINGS

The ceiling you'll probably use will be made up of panels of a mineral material that are suspended by a metal framework from the roof or from the floor above. The least expensive type to use is the *lay-in* ceiling. A grid of metal supports is hung and ceiling panels that fit the square or rectangular openings are dropped in to rest on the exposed grid (see Figure 41-1). More expensive is the recessed grid in which the panels are suspended below the framework by about three-quarters of an inch. A *spline* or concealed suspension ceiling is still more attractive and more costly. Here the suspension system is completely hidden by the panels.

In addition to cost, your ceilings will be chosen on the basis of your need for access to the space above the ceiling, on fire code requirements, appearance, and on your acoustic needs. The panels come in many different sizes and patterns. Discuss them with your architect.

In some types of construction, the tops of the partitions must be supported by the ceiling grid. This may restrict where you can place your partitions.

DOORS

Doors will be needed to close off many rooms in your office for visual and acoustic privacy. Hinged doors, the type used most frequently, have one major drawback: The swing of the door projects into the room—or worse, out into a hallway. In a small treatment room, this may consume space critically needed for equipment or for the room's occupants.

To avoid this problem, you may have to consider sliding (pocket) doors that are attached to a track above the door frame. They are more expensive to install than hinged doors, but, when opened, they slide out of sight into a recess in the door frame. The principal difficulty with them is their tendency to bind unless top-quality track hardware is used and unless the frame is carefully made with adequate clearance on both sides of the door.

In addition to the choice of hinged versus sliding, doors come in many woods (metal doors are used primarily for fire retardation, which is beyond the scope of this discussion) and in several basic types, including solid-core, hollow-core, panel, carved, folding, and louver.

Hollow-core doors are made of two thin sheets of plywood glued to wooden spacers around the perimeter of the sheets. The door then looks solid, but except for wood blocks where hardware is to be installed, the inner portion is empty.

Solid-core doors are made of wood all the way through. Solid doors cost more than the hollow ones, but they cut sound transmission much more, especially if they are well fitted. I recommend them. They also retard fire better than hollow doors.

Use louver doors on coat closets. They permit air circulation, which dries wet garments and avoids odors (see Figure 41-2).

FLOORS

The architect may ask what type of floor coverings you intend to use, because your choice will determine how the underlying floor is to be prepared. For example, if you are converting an old house, the hardwood floors may be irregular and not quite flat. This can be a serious problem if you intend to cover them with sheet vinyl or vinyl asbestos tile. Before either of these *resilient* floor coverings is installed, the builder will have to cover the old floors with an *underlayment*, a layer of plywood or composition board or a leveling compound that can be made smooth and flat.

On the other hand, if the old floors are to be covered by carpeting, the padding under the carpet will compensate for most of the floors' irregularities and no special preparation may be needed.

Now is the time, too, to let the architect know if you are planning to use any extremely heavy equipment that could require reinforcement of the floor. An example is a filing system in which several shelf files are grouped on tracks and rolled apart for access.

22
ELEVATIONS, WINDOWS, AND LANDSCAPING: THE VIEW FROM OUTSIDE

The first drawings of the exterior of your building will probably be perspective sketches that incorporate the points discussed at your early meetings with the architect. A cardboard model will help if the architect is willing to make one.

ELEVATIONS

Has the architect caught the spirit of what you are after? Has he brought in ideas that are new to you? Don't jump to a snap decision. Think about the designs for a few days. As you do, consider these points:

☐ Does the building look like it belongs on this site? In this neighborhood?

☐ Is the front entry one you'll be proud to walk through?

☐ Does the building project the image you want to be identified with?

☐ Will patients feel comfortable coming to this building?

☐ Are the proportions of the building harmonious?

☐ Do the roof, walls, windows, and doors give the appearance of belonging with each other?

Now is the time to look long and critically at these points, as soon as the drawings become detailed enough to permit it.

If the job is one of renovating and adding to an existing building—as ours was—the blending of new and old increases the difficulty. To keep costs down, you should make as few changes as possible, yet the new portion should not look tacked on to the old.

The materials used for the exterior of office buildings vary so much that I won't attempt to discuss them. Choose a material that will be attractive for a long period with minimum maintenance and that conforms to local building and fire codes. Your architect is your best guide here.

WINDOWS

Windows are important elements in your building for several reasons:

☐ Their size, shape, and number can enhance or diminish the attractiveness of the structure from both outside and inside.

☐ They permit maximum appreciation of a pleasing view.

☐ Most people feel more comfortable in rooms with windows than in windowless rooms.

☐ Windows are areas of heat transfer, which can mean significant increases in energy costs for heating and air conditioning if the windows are of poor quality or poorly installed.

☐ They are expensive. Depending on the material used for the frame, the number of glass panels in each sash, the style of window (casement, double-hung, awning, for example), and the overall quality, a window may cost more than twice as much as the area of blank wall that it replaces.

Your architect must weigh carefully these opposing concerns. He'll have to select windows that provide light, but that, especially on the ground floor, are placed to allow privacy and security. More windows mean more natural light and, generally, a more attractive interior and exterior, but they also mean higher initial expense for the windows and for shades, drapes, or blinds, increased energy costs, and increased maintenance.

We've been pleased with the special type of casement window that was installed in the new portion of our building. Between an inner removable storm sash and an outer fixed sash are thin venetian blinds that can be adjusted from inside the room. Since the blinds are between two layers of glass, they seldom need dusting and they eliminate the need for shades, drapes, or curtains for privacy and for control of sunlight (see Figure 41-5).

LANDSCAPING

Since landscaping materials and techniques are important and since they vary greatly in different parts of the country, you should give some thought at an early stage to the planning of your building's surroundings. While your architect will specify how the land is to be graded for drainage, he may not consider that landscape design is also his responsibility. Ask him. You could need a landscape architect as well.

You'll want attractive trees, shrubs, and other plantings to enhance the appearance of your building. It makes little sense to spend large sums on the building and then to surround it with a barren parking lot.

Imaginative use of landscaping materials can do many things: Their beauty improves staff morale and lessens patients' tensions. They can block out an objectionable view or frame an attractive one. They can serve as sound insulators if nearby traffic noises are oppressive. In the northern part of the country, evergreen trees on the north side of a building can be a partial barrier to winter winds, thereby keeping your fuel bills down. Deciduous trees south of the building can provide welcome shade in the summer, while allowing the winter sun to filter through their bare branches, once again aiding your energy conservation efforts. See Chapter 26 for detailed suggestions about using plants to save energy.

Try to go first class in the quality of plants. Inexpensive plants are usually cheap because they were not properly cared for in the nursery. They're no bargain if they're dead within a year. A reliable nurseryman should be able to guide you in this and in other areas of exterior design.

The cost of site work (grading, paving, landscaping) usually ranges from 3-5 percent or more of the building's total cost, but the landscaping part of that figure varies with the site.

Try to have your landscape plan completed before the final grading of the property is done. This avoids the need for additional earth moving at a later date.

23
REVISIONS

Preparation of each set of drawings is followed by a meeting with the architect, at which the good and bad points are discussed. The architect makes notes on the basis of which he'll later alter the drawings. Be sure to tell him which dimensions must not be changed. For example, if you want your lab to be six inches wider than shown, tell this to the architect, but let him know also that it must not be at the expense of the room next to the lab. When each new set of plans arrives, check any critical dimensions carefully.

Don't assume that a room's size remains unchanged from one set of drawings to the next, merely because you did not ask for any alteration in it. The changes in the plans may be made by a draftsman who wasn't present at your meeting with the architect. He may have to work solely from the latter's notes. Mistakes happen. Catch them early!

Study each set of drawings carefully and try to visualize how the office will work. Properly scaled outlines of furniture and equipment will be invaluable.

Once your room layout is complete and you're satisfied with it, don't tamper with the plan unless it's obvious that something important was missed earlier. As the plans become more detailed, particularly once mechanical features are added, each subsequent change in a wall's location may require a whole series of other changes; a chain reaction occurs, which can have effects in locations remote from the point of change. Of course, if the change is important, do it. Otherwise, you'll be kicking yourself for the next 20 years.

If you're putting up a building, the same principles apply, but there are other concerns as well. If there are several owner-tenants, the desirability of each suite has to be carefully considered or you'll have some disgruntled partners later. The earlier you settle this problem, the better.

Ideally, all office plans should be completed at the same time as the building plans are, so that construction can proceed at the most rapid rate. This rarely happens, but it's worth aiming for.

V
MECHANICAL ASPECTS OF YOUR OFFICE

24
YOUR ELECTRICAL NEEDS

While your floor plan and the traffic flow it dictates are important for the efficient operation of your office, the mechanical features can make your workday comfortable or irritating. Poorly placed lighting, an electrical outlet in the wrong location, a sink too high or too low, an inadequate intercom or telephone arrangement: Each will bother you whenever you use it. Each is preventable. The material in Section V will focus your attention on the details that should concern you at this stage.

The architect will prepare an electrical plan for your office. This will be a copy of your floor plan to which he has added symbols that explain to the electrician what is needed. The plan will be based on the architect's understanding of your needs, so be clear when you explain them.

A brief review of how electric power gets to where you need it is an appropriate way to start this discussion. The utility company's heavy wires carry power to the electric *service entrance* of the building. The wires pass through the wall to the building's basement or utility room. If there are several office suites, the incoming power lines will supply current to each through its own meter. A separate meter measures current used by the building itself for lobby, hallway, and exterior lighting, operation of heating equipment, and other functions not related to one specific office. These are discussed separately in this chapter.

From the meter, the power for your office goes next to a control box called a *breaker panel.* It contains a series of circuit breakers, each of which has a rated capacity, such as 15 or 20 amperes. If the current flow through a circuit exceeds that capacity, as in an overloaded or a short circuit, the breaker opens (interrupts the current), thereby preventing a fire.

When your office is wired, the electrician will run wires for every circuit from the breaker panel. There are certain standard sizes and capacities for these wires required by the electrical code. He knows, for example, that not more than 1,200 watts of lighting fixtures should be on a 15-ampere circuit.

When the architect prepares your electrical plan, he won't specify how many of these general circuits are to be used. The plan will show the number, size, and placement of lighting fixtures and the location of duplex wall outlets. It will be up to the electrician to work out the number of circuits needed for these purposes.

The architect will also identify on the plan those pieces of equipment that require their own separate circuits, sometimes called *dedicated* circuits. These will be items that require large amounts of current, such as a dental chair, an examining table, or an X-ray machine, and also those that need different voltages, such as a central suction unit or central air conditioner, which may use 230 volts rather than 115.

MASTER ELECTRICAL SHUT-OFF

Early in the planning process, you must decide if you want a *master shut-off* in your office. This extremely useful device disconnects all electrical circuits in your office by the flipping of a single switch except for those—listed below—that must remain on. It eliminates any chance of damage to a piece of equipment from being left on overnight or over a weekend, and it eliminates the need to go from room to room turning off lights and apparatus.

If you want this convenience, and I recommend it, be prepared to spend an extra $400 to $600 or more, depending on your office size. Your architect will specify it on the electrical plan, and he will list those items that are *not* to be connected to the shut-off. Any circuit not on this list is to be disconnected by the shut-off switch. This switch should be in a convenient location, but where it cannot be tripped accidentally or by a curious patient (inside a closet is a good spot).

In our office the following are *not* operated by the master shut-off:

☐ Entry-exit lighting to find our way from the shut-off switch to the office door when leaving at night. Only one or two hallway lights are needed. We turn them off separately as we leave.

☐ Heating (which is controlled by a clock thermostat), ventilating, and air-conditioning equipment.

☐ Burglar- and fire-alarm circuits.

☐ Outlet for telephones. If your phones are supplied by the telephone company, they'll be on the company's power, which is unrelated to the office's electrical system. But if you buy a telephone system, as discussed in Chapter 28, your phones must be on office power, which must be on all the time. Otherwise, your phones will be dead when you turn off the master shut-off switch and you'll get no messages to your answering machine or answering service.

☐ Outlet for telephone-answering machine.

☐ Refrigerator outlet.

☐ Emergency-lighting outlets, into which are plugged small light units that turn on automatically in a power failure. Specify that these outlets are to be up near the ceiling so that the emergency lights won't be accidentally bumped. Other items you might want to include in this list for your office are:

☐ Electric-clock outlets. We don't have these. We use battery-operated clocks.

☐ Heating devices, such as incubators for cultures.

☐ Entry doorbell.

☐ Any other special equipment that must be on at all times.

DUPLEX OUTLETS

The electrical plan will show wall outlets—also called duplex receptacles—spaced at intervals around each room. Where no height is specified, the electrician will place them about 12 inches up on the wall, but you can have them at any height you want. Just tell the architect. Examine the location of these outlets carefully on the plan. Consider them in relation to the furniture, lamps, or equipment that must be plugged into them. Proper placement and adequate numbers of outlets will avoid unsightly and dangerous trailing wires. Extra outlets are an inexpensive one-time expense.

If the exact height of an outlet is critical, the plan should state whether the specified height refers to the center or to the bottom of the outlet box.

Electricians usually install these outlets vertically, but if you want them horizontal (receptacles side by side instead of one above the other) have this noted on the plan.

Office equipment that should have outlets immediately adjacent to them to avoid trailing wires include:

- [ ] electric typewriter(s);
- [ ] copying machine;
- [ ] calculator;
- [ ] telephone-answering machine;
- [ ] pencil sharpener;
- [ ] postage meter;
- [ ] computer.

For example, if the electric typewriter's countertop is to be about 26 inches high, have an outlet placed 29 inches *AFF* (above the finished floor). This will provide an outlet about three inches above the countertop on the wall behind the machine. A neat alternative, which keeps the wire almost completely out of sight, is this: Order the outlet at 20 inches AFF. This will place it just below the countertop. Later, have a hole drilled in the counter, large enough for the typewriter's plug and wire to pass through to the outlet underneath.

For each piece of special electrical equipment, the architect should indicate on the electrical plan or in attached notes how and where the wires to that item are to terminate for connection when your equipment is installed. You'll have to get this information from your equipment dealer. He should supply a manufacturer's template with the needed information. Switch locations for this equipment may also be required.

For some switches, you may want a pilot light in the hall to signal that a particular room or piece of equipment is in use. For example, when the safelight in our darkroom is switched on, a red pilot light goes on in the hall. Also, each X-ray machine is turned on and off by a switch in the hall that has its own accompanying pilot light (see Figure 61-2). This lessens the chance of a machine being accidentally left on for a long period.

You've undoubtedly noticed by this time that in order to plan properly for your electrical needs you must make decisions about furniture, equipment, and cabinetwork at a much earlier stage than you may have thought. This has several benefits: It will spur you to choose and to order these items with adequate time for delivery, even allowing for the inevitable delays. Also, it will prevent the anxiety and much greater expense of suddenly recognizing the need for extra outlets or special circuits when the office is nearly finished.

LIGHTING THE OFFICE

The kind of lighting you use and its intensity will have an effect on everyone in your office. Experts concerned with eye comfort offer these principles for lighting the office:

1. The more detailed a task, the more illumination is needed. A waiting room, where patients casually glance through magazines, does not need the same brightness level as your secretary's desk.

2. *Ambient* lighting, the general light level in a room, should not be markedly less than the *task* lighting, the illumination of the work surface. The task-brightness to ambient-brightness ratio should probably not be greater than five to one, and some authorities suggest three to one as the limit. Increasing the brightness of the room in relation to the brightness of the work surface improves visual efficiency. If there is a marked contrast between the two, fatigue and strain usually result.

3. Lighting needs increase with age. As we get older, we need more light to maintain the same level of vision. A 50-year-old secretary needs brighter desk lighting than a 25-year-old.

4. Shiny, highly polished desk surfaces reflect light as glare, causing discomfort and reducing efficiency.

5. Light-colored walls and floor coverings can increase room brightness by 35 percent or more, reducing the need for artificial lighting.

6. Placement of ceiling fixtures can be critical over a desk or other work surface. The fixture should be placed so that the shadow of the person working there will not be cast on the work. It must also be positioned to minimize *veiling* *reflection.* This is the image of the light source bouncing off the task (such as a printed page) into the eyes of the worker.

7. For each watt of energy used you will get approximately *four* times as much light from fluorescent lamps as from incandescent lamps. In addition to saving energy, fluorescent lamps require less frequent replacement. In places where you must use incandescent lighting, consider installing solid-state dimmer switches for energy savings and brightness control.

8. Indirect lighting, which means light from a hidden source, is useful where quiet uniform illumination is preferred. It should be considered for hallways and for places where soft lighting is needed. It's not adequate for most tasks.

Here is how we handled the lighting needs in different parts of our office:

Waiting room. Our architect designed indirect fluorescent strip lighting supplemented by "high hat" incandescents (see Figure 41-1). Illumination is varied. Part of the room has subdued lighting, while other areas are comfortable for reading or filling out insurance forms.

Business office. We wanted comfortable desk levels for bookkeeping, recording appointments, and other detail work. Our receptionist's and insurance clerk's work areas are lit by two fluorescent fixtures, each with four 40-watt tubes. This produces about 50 to 80 foot candles of illumination at desk height. The receptionist has an additional fluorescent strip under the pigeon holes above her desk (see Figures 41-2, 41-3).

Halls. Our main concern is to avoid shadows and to light the floor evenly. We use fluorescent lighting covered by a light cove. A skylight adds natural daylight to the central hallway (Figure 24-1). Other hall areas have recessed "high-hat" ceiling fixtures, four feet apart, with 75-watt reflector flood bulbs.

Exam/treatment rooms. Each of our treatment rooms, which average nine and one-half by 11 feet, has two fluorescent ceiling fixtures, each of which has four 40-watt tubes. This is supplemented by window light in the daytime.

If you use cool-white fluorescent tubes, eight such lamps should provide adequate ambient light in your treatment room. But if you intend to use the kind of tubes that imitate natural light—their color temperature is 5,000 to 6,000° K—you'll need more of them. Each such tube emits only about 70 percent as much light as a cool-white lamp of similar wattage.

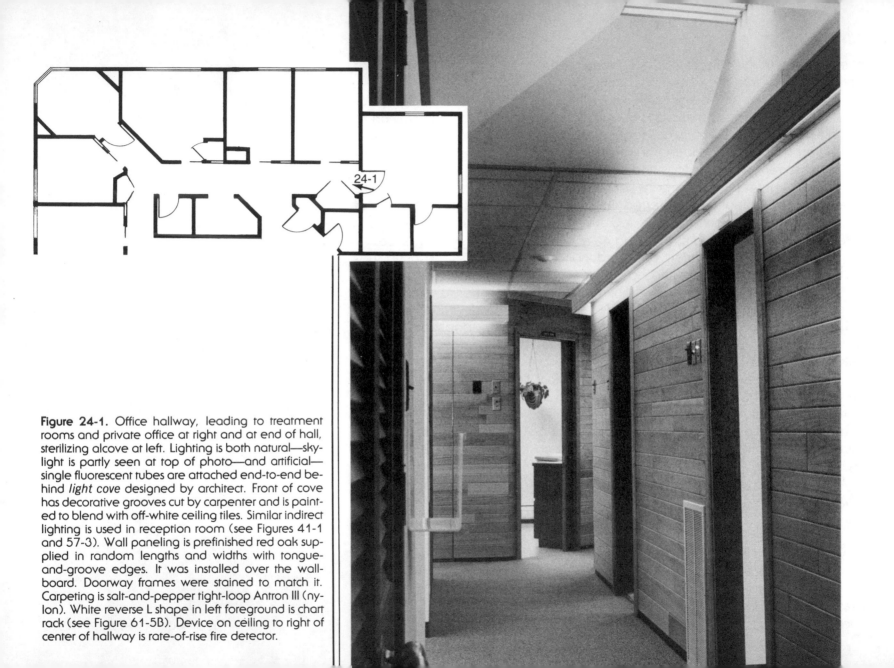

Figure 24-1. Office hallway, leading to treatment rooms and private office at right and at end of hall, sterilizing alcove at left. Lighting is both natural—skylight is partly seen at top of photo—and artificial—single fluorescent tubes are attached end-to-end behind *light cove* designed by architect. Front of cove has decorative grooves cut by carpenter and is painted to blend with off-white ceiling tiles. Similar indirect lighting is used in reception room (see Figures 41-1 and 57-3). Wall paneling is prefinished red oak supplied in random lengths and widths with tongue-and-groove edges. It was installed over the wallboard. Doorway frames were stained to match it. Carpeting is salt-and-pepper tight-loop Antron III (nylon). White reverse L shape in left foreground is chart rack (see Figure 61-5B). Device on ceiling to right of center of hallway is rate-of-rise fire detector.

Consultation room/private office. The amount of illumination here depends on whether you use this area primarily as a workroom for reading and writing or as a place for discussions with patients. We use it mainly as a workroom. Our 11½ × 14-foot office has two four-tube (40 watts/tube) fixtures.

Laboratory and sterilization areas. These work areas require bright lighting. Our sterilization and central-supply alcove, which is only about 35 square feet, has 160 watts of fluorescent lighting.

Lavatories. We find that diffused fluorescent lighting is desirable above the mirror over the sink. A single 24-inch tube is adequate.

Storage and utility areas. Every closet, except the shallowest, has its own ceiling fixture. This lighting is especially important for our walk-in supply closet where an assistant may have to read small labels on stored items.

Basement storage areas. These are well lit for three reasons:

☐ ease of storing and finding items left there;

☐ servicing of equipment; and

☐ security: It reassures timid staff members that no one is lurking in gloomy shadows. Our basement is lit by many single-tube fluorescents.

Your architect should offer suggestions about the type, size, and number of lighting fixtures. Insist on seeing pictures of each recommended type to be sure that you like its appearance and that it can be coordinated with your decorating scheme. In general, if there is doubt about whether an additional fixture is needed for an area, put it in. Adding it later will be messy and expensive.

This is also a good time to decide if you will need special lighting for plants in the office. Many plants do well with window light or under the fluorescents used for general room lighting, but some need special light sources.

Check carefully where the architect has indicated all light switches on the electrical plan. You may want "three-way" switches in some locations to control a fixture from either of two places. In areas with several fixtures, decide if you want the flexibility of turning on some fixtures, but not others.

Electricians usually install these switches 48 inches above the floor, which most adults find a comfortable height. If you want a switch placed lower, as in a lavatory to be used mostly by children, or higher, to keep a particular switch out of the reach of children, tell the architect about it at this stage.

LOW-VOLTAGE CIRCUITS

All of the office's electrical requirements mentioned so far involve 110- to 120-volt (or higher) lines. The electricians will install either armored ("BX") or plastic covered ("Romex") cable for them depending on local code requirements.

There is another kind of wiring that must also be installed. The voltages are generally lower than 30 volts, which means that much lighter wires are used. These low-voltage circuits involve many different systems. Some of them may be wired by the electricians, whereas for others, different installers will be needed. Below is a list of the low-voltage systems in our office. The number in parentheses indicates the chapter in which each is described.

☐ alarms: burglar (31), fire (31), and water (61);
☐ annunciator (61);
☐ door-latch release (31);
☐ intercom (29);
☐ music system (32);
☐ signal system (29, 61); and
☐ telephones (28).

THE BUILDING'S ELECTRICAL NEEDS

The electrical plan for the building—as distinct from an individual office—includes the location and capacity of the wiring needed for:

☐ heating equipment;
☐ air-conditioning and ventilating equipment;
☐ thermostats;
☐ lobby, hallway, utility-room lighting;
☐ elevator(s);
☐ exterior lighting;
☐ controls for exterior lighting—usually a timer switch or a photoelectric switch;
☐ wall outlets for hallways and lobby (for use of vacuum cleaners, other maintenance equipment);
☐ emergency lighting; and
☐ alarm systems.

LIGHTING THE BUILDING

Your architect will specify interior light fixtures for lobby, hallways, and common storage and utility areas based on the principles mentioned earlier in this chapter. In addition, he'll plan for lights identifying all of the building's exits.

Exterior lighting should be carefully considered for several reasons:

Security. Well-lit perimeter lighting reduces nighttime burglaries; patients with appointments after dark feel safer in a well-lit parking area.

Accident prevention. Illumination of walks, ramps, and curbs reduces chances of falls on slippery wet surfaces.

Attractiveness. Properly placed exterior lighting can enhance the beauty of your building.

To keep energy costs down, the architect will have to plan the location of these fixtures carefully. There are too many types for me to discuss them all, but a few principles are worth mentioning:

1. Exterior lighting generally should be well diffused. If the light source is bright and has no diffuser, it should be placed high enough on the building or on a pole so that it doesn't shine uncomfortably in the eyes of persons walking or driving near your building.

2. All parts of the parking area should be equally well lit to avoid menacing shadows.

3. All doorways should be brightly lit for security and for ease in locking and unlocking the door.

4. The size and shape of fixtures and poles should be in harmony with the building and its surroundings. Ask for pictures or, better still, samples of the fixtures suggested.

5. Your exterior lighting should be switched on and off automatically by a timer switch or by a photoelectric switch if you want these lights on all night.

6. Find out if your local utility company will rent poles and fixtures to you and provide power for a flat amount per month. Sometimes, this is less costly than buying and installing your own.

7. The lamps used in some outside fixtures are not stocked in local hardware stores. Order several extras when the fixtures are ordered. Be sure to specify long-life lamps for use in fixtures that are difficult to reach.

25
PLUMBING

You will have to tell the architect what you need and want with regard to plumbing in your office and building.

THE OFFICE'S PLUMBING NEEDS

The following list will alert you to the topics you should think about:

Water filters. Ask the water company about particulate matter in the water supply. Some professional equipment, such as dental turbines, can be damaged by suspended matter in the water line. A filter may be needed for this or for elimination of a bad taste. Find out from your equipment-supply company if you should have one installed as protection for the equipment you're buying.

Water pressure. The water utility can also tell you about the pressure in the water line. Too high a pressure can damage sensitive equipment. A pressure reducer is the solution. Again, your supplier or plumber can advise you.

Hot-water supply. Most buildings are supplied by a central hot-water heater, but in some medical-dental buildings, each suite provides its own hot water. If you are to supply your own, be sure its size is adequate, particularly if you have many uses for hot water. These include handwashing, instrument scrubbing, maintenance of X-ray developer temperature, even a shower in your private lavatory. A 10-gallon tank would probably be ample, but ask your architect's opinion. A gas-fired heater is likely to be the cheapest to operate, but if gas isn't available you'll have to use electricity. Insist that the hot-water heater and hot-water pipes be insulated for energy conservation and to prevent burns. The insulation around the pipes should have arrows showing the direction of the water flow. If you need hot water only at one or two sinks and the building doesn't supply it, consider using an ''instant'' hot-water appliance. This will avoid the need for both the heater and the pipes.

Mixing valves. In some situations, you may find it desirable to have the plumber install a mixing valve to deliver water at a preset temperature to a piece of equipment. For example, since we wanted lukewarm water for our patients to rinse with, and since our new dental units didn't have self-contained heaters, we had a mixing valve placed in the water lines to these treatment rooms. It provides water to the units at a comfortable temperature. Patients with sensitive teeth appreciate this. Another, more expensive, solution to this problem is to provide a separate special heater for each unit.

Master water shut-off. If you will have water lines running to equipment in many rooms, you should have a master water shut-off installed in the same location as the master electrical shut-off. The plumber can bring the hot and cold lines to this location and install valves. Get the type that is operated by a quarter-turn of a lever (see Figure 49-1, D).

Sinks. The three materials you are most likely to consider for sinks in your treatment rooms, lab, sterilizing areas, and other rooms are stainless steel, vitreous china, and porcelain (actually cast iron or steel with heavy porcelain baked on).

Despite its _____ n used for a sink. Dried water _____ For this reason, I suggest using _____ om and lavatory sinks. Vitreous _____ ereas porcelain is usually specifi__

In work roo__ _____ , however, stainless steel is de__ _____ ment is dropped on it, but stai__ _____ rks on it won't be seen by patie__

If your sinks _____ ow high you want them. Standa__ _____ ches, but if you're short or tall, another height may be better for you. If your sinks are to be mounted in countertops, the countertop height will determine sink height. We'll have more to say about that in Chapter 42.

Be sure you get your work sinks deep enough. Standard sink depths are six or seven and one-half inches, but you'll find 10- or even 12-inch depths useful if many soiled instruments have to soak, or if large items, such as X-ray developer tanks or processor racks, have to be cleaned.

If you use plaster in any of your work, as in an orthopedic or a dental practice, be sure to have a plaster trap installed to avoid clogged drain lines.

The interior dimensions of our sinks are:

	Length (side to side)	Width (front to back)	Depth
Treatment rooms (porcelain):	15½''	9½''	6''
Sterilizing area (stainless):	19''	16''	10''
Darkroom (stainless):	12''	9½''	7½''

Lavatory sinks can be the wall-hung vitreous-china type, but there are several attractive and inexpensive alternatives. One is a combined sink and counter made of a synthetic marble, which is sold with its own cabinet underneath. The cabinet hides the pipes, and it's a convenient storage place.

We bought such units for our two lavatories at a local discount store, and we are quite satisfied with them. If you decide to do this, too, just be sure that the construction contract calls for the plumber to install these sinks as well as any that he supplies. If it's not in the contract you can be sure that you'll be billed for it as an "extra."

One problem with the cabinet plus sink in the lavatory is that its interior is one more thing that must be cleaned. Also, in a small lavatory, the cabinet may make the room feel even smaller.

Another alternative is an imitation marble sink with an apron that extends down in front to hide the pipes.

Faucet controls. There are at least four basic types of faucet controls for you to choose from: separate knobs for hot and cold water, single-lever controls, foot controls, and automatic electronic controls.

Either separate knobs or single levers are fine for lavatory or workroom sinks. For your treatment rooms, you'll probably choose either single levers (operated by hand, wrist, or elbow) or foot controls. We chose foot controls. They are more expensive, an extra $50 or more per sink, but we like the convenience they offer. This is purely a matter of personal preference. Much more expensive are the electronic controls. The movement of your hands into the sink breaks a light beam that starts the water flowing.

If you choose foot controls, be sure the architect specifies where the pedals are to be placed in relation to the center of the sink. They should be slightly to the left or right but not exactly in the center. At our sinks, the midpoint between the hot and cold pedals is four inches to the right of the sink's center. This puts the pedals in a convenient position for my right to control them as I stand at the sink.

Toilets. These can range from the simplest type required by your plumbing code to elaborate models. The type that is hung on the wall, while quite expensive, makes cleaning easier in the lavatory. Ours are floor models with no frills. Your local plumbing code may require a certain type or a minimum size of seat for the patients' lavatory.

Gas. If gas is available in the building, you may wish to have it installed for use in your lab and/or your treatment rooms. Before you do, however, ask yourself if your needs can be satisfied instead with small containers of butane or propane. This can save a substantial amount in plumbing costs. But don't do it if it will mean frequent inconvenience for you or your staff.

Compressed air. This is essential for all modern dental offices and for some medical suites as well. The compressor you choose should have the following features:

☐ Adequate horsepower, air volume, and pressure. These, in turn, depend on the number of rooms to be supplied. Ask your supplier.

☐ Most economical voltage—230 volts sometimes provides an energy saving.

☐ Dryer, either built-in or added, to prevent moisture from damaging your equipment.

☐ Backup capacity. Get a model that is really two compressors joined together. You'll generally need only one at a time, but the second is a valuable standby for use when the first is out of order. Use them alternately, so that each is run regularly.

Central suction. There are two basic types of central suction units: The *high-air-volume* type is a turbine that moves large quantities of air. This is needed when large quantities of liquid must be picked up, but it doesn't provide the kind of high vacuum needed for surgical aspiration. In fact, such a unit may require air passage over the motor to cool it. If you try to use one for a long period with a small aspirator tip and no other open port to admit air, you are likely to overheat and burn out the motor.

The *high-vacuum* (sometimes called *high-mercury)* type is essentially an impellor pump that delivers the kind of suction needed for surgical aspiration. We use this type in our periodontal practice.

Regardless of which type is better for you, the following principles apply:

1. Have a backup! Ours is two pumps on a single frame. We can use either or both.

2. Use 208 or higher voltage if it's available. Since the suction equipment may run most of the day, the higher voltage is more energy efficient. If three-phase current is available this, too, will often result in energy savings. You may need a special transformer, called a *buck-and-boost* transformer, if your line voltage is not up to the required level. Our line delivers 208 volts, which is boosted by the transformer to the 230 volts needed by the motors.

3. Your system will probably have a low-voltage switch in each treatment room to turn the central suction on and off. However, most central-suction units are rated for continuous duty, which means that they can remain on for hours at a time. ·

4. Try to have the suction unit in the building's basement or at the lowest possible level. The higher the pump or turbine is located, the harder it must work to pull liquids uphill.

5. The central suction unit will empty into the building's waste line, but the manner of this connection will vary, depending on the type of unit and on the local plumbing code. If a scavenging mask is used for nitrous-oxide/oxygen analgesia, your suction system will have to be vented to the outside of the building. You may also have to vent the system to keep the system's odors from re-entering the office. Your plumber and/or equipment supplier will have to check this with the building inspector.

6. Some impellor (pump)-type suction units require a continuous flow of water to maintain the suction seal. If yours is this type, you'll have to be careful that the pump is always turned off *before* the office's water supply is cut off for some plumbing repair. Such a pump burns out if it runs without a flow of water. At least one model of this type recirculates some of this water, thereby reducing water consumption.

Anesthetic gases. The installation of nitrous-oxide/oxygen central systems has been subjected to increasingly strict controls in recent years. This has occurred because of the discovery of health hazards from prolonged exposure to low levels of nitrous-oxide and because of the incidence of serious fires in this kind of equipment.

Your equipment dealer should be able to supply your architect with the specific installation requirements for your area. If there's any doubt, the local building inspector should be consulted in advance. Your architect should make these requirements a part of the plumbing plan, so that the plumber knows what will be expected. Some of these regulations include use of continuous lengths of a special grade of copper tubing, severe pressure testing of the completed system, an alarm to alert the office to a low-pressure condition, and an exhaust fan where tanks are stored.

HOW WILL THE LINES BE INSTALLED?

Placement of your plumbing lines depends on the type of building and your office's location in it. Here are some of the possibilities:

1. Ground floor above a basement: Pipes run along the ceiling of the basement. Noisy equipment—compressor, suction—can be kept there as well.

2. Ground floor in existing building on slab, no basement: Channels are cut through slab, and pipes rest in the earth under the slab. They are covered with sand for protection. Then the concrete slab is patched and smoothed to prepare it for your floor covering.

3. Second—or higher—floor: Holes are bored in the floor and the pipes are run in the space between your floor and the dropped ceiling of the suite below.

There are other ways plumbing can be installed, such as under false floors or by means of umbilicals from a piece of equipment to the wall.

A most important consideration, wherever your plumbing lines are located, is that all waste lines have accessible *clean-outs:* threaded plugs that can be unscrewed to clear the pipe if it's clogged.

THE BUILDING'S PLUMBING NEEDS

Your architect or his engineer will decide on the sizes of water supply and waste lines for your building and the distribution of these lines to individual offices. He'll also specify the size of the hot-water heater and of other centrally placed equipment.

It may prevent headaches at some time in the future if the building's specifications require that when the building is finished, the contractor is to submit a floor plan that shows the location of all major pipes and ducts and the direction of flow in each.

There are some plumbing needs in the building that do not involve individual offices. These include public lavatories, janitors' sinks, and outside hose bibbs (faucets). I suggest that if your building is in a region where winter temperatures often drop well below freezing you should ask the architect to specify *freeze-proof bibbs*. Such a faucet has a long stem with the valve located inside the building's wall. Its advantage—worth the extra cost—is that it's not necessary to drain the faucet each year in the fall. Since your building will probably not have a full-time maintenance person, this becomes one less annual chore to worry about.

26
HEATING, VENTILATING, AND AIR CONDITIONING; ENERGY CONSERVATION

Unless you own the building in which your office is located you will probably not have much control over the heating, ventilating, and air-conditioning systems (HVAC). As noted elsewhere, you should investigate the adequacy of the indoor climate control before renting or buying space in any building.

OFFICE HVAC

Many patients visiting a medical or dental office are anxious. Any feeling of overheating or of being chilled may be interpreted by the patient as a product of his own fear.

In order to keep comfortable temperature levels, you should have several zones. The concern here is related to the direction your windows face and the temperature needs of interior versus exterior rooms. If your office has windows that face several exposures, as ours does, the air conditioning may be designed to separate the cooling of the eastern rooms from those facing west. Your architect or his engineer will work this out if some flexibility is available. Of course, if you are putting up the structure you should make known what you prefer with regard to office temperature.

If you're a physician who treats many elderly patients or whose patients must undress, you'll want your treatment rooms to be several degrees warmer than the rest of the office. This can be accomplished in several ways:

☐ a separate heating zone can be provided for those rooms;

☐ a small adjustable thermostat may be installed on each baseboard radiation unit (if circulating hot-water heat is used); or

☐ a supplementary radiation unit, such as a built-in electric heater, can be placed in the wall of each treatment room.

If the HVAC system is a good one, it will also have provision for circulating the air in the office and introducing outside air, even in the winter. Household-type recirculating central air-conditioning systems usually are single zone and don't provide for admission of clean air. They rely instead on air seepage around windows and doors for the addition of fresh air. Some medical buildings, especially those built at the lowest possible cost, place a single household-type central unit in each office. Such a system is likely to be inadequate for your needs in terms of adjustability, sound control, and flexibility for future changes. Avoid it.

If you have provision for bringing in fresh air, your system will probably have a motorized damper that will allow outside air to be mixed with the office's air. Be sure that such a unit has a "limit switch" that will close the damper before the warmed or cooled inside air is excessively diluted by the air from outside. Otherwise, your fuel bills will go up.

Some parts of your office can be sources of hazardous gases or unpleasant odors, or are interior rooms with no outside ventilation. Such areas need exhaust fans, which should be noted on the electrical, HVAC, and plumbing plans. The electrician will have to supply an outlet at or near the ceiling for the fan motor, while another tradesman—a plumber or duct man—installs the pipe that carries the exhausted air to the outside or to a ventilating stack in the interior of a large building.

Examples of areas where exhaust fans might be used are: lavatories, sterilizing area, darkroom, lab, and tank-storage closet (for anesthetic gases). The sterilizing area will also need a special venting system if ethylene oxide gas sterilization is used.

The darkroom presents a slight additional problem: The door must be tight-fitting at all its edges to exclude light, but doing this also reduces air passage. An exhaust fan is likely to be ineffective or to overheat in such a situation. To solve this problem, get a lightproof louver, which admits air but not light, from your equipment supplier for installation in the darkroom door.

A checklist of energy-saving measures for your office can be found in Chapter 60. During your planning stage, you should be aware of these points:

1. Exhaust fans should comply with the energy code and not remove too much of your heated or cooled air.

2. Thermostats must be placed where they will not be affected by sunlight, drafts, or heat-producing apparatus.

In most office air-conditioning systems, each room has a *feed* duct that brings cooled air to the room. The air it replaces moves out into the hall to a *return* duct that carries it back to the blower unit. Usually the gap at the bottom of the door to the room is sufficient to allow this air out even when the door is closed. However, if you have a room for which maximum soundproofing is required, the door in that room must fit tightly, with no gaps. For optimum ventilation, it's desirable for such a room to have its own air-conditioning return duct, but be prepared to pay extra for it.

BUILDING HVAC

The heating, ventilating, and air conditioning for your building will be worked out by your architect and his engineer, but be sure to make your ideas known about the kind of temperature control you need.

A frequently overlooked point is that basement storage areas must be adequately heated to prevent damage to stored records and supplies and for the comfort of the people who use them.

Both the shortage and the high price of energy make the selection of fuel and equipment critical to the efficient and profitable operation of your building. But don't let an urge to save money on energy cause you to skimp on heating or cooling equipment. If you do you'll be constantly irritated by uncomfortable temperatures in your own office, and you'll find other tenants besieging you with complaints.

The following checklist of measures that can aid your energy-conservation efforts was developed by the Council on Dental Practice of the American Dental Association, published September 17, 1979, in *ADA News*.

☐ Proper insulation can reduce heating and cooling loads by as much as 20 and 30 percent.

☐ Adequate caulking and weatherstripping can save another 10 percent.

☐ Older buildings without thermal glass need storm windows.

☐ Heat pumps, helpful in some heating and cooling systems, make use of the temperature outside the building. Ask your architect if they can be used in your building.

☐ Select air-conditioning units with the highest efficiency ratings.

☐ Have water-heater thermostat set at lowest suitable temperature.

Other energy-saving methods listed by the *ADA News* can be found in Chapter 60, in the discussion of office maintenance.

In our renovated building, we approached the problem of reducing heat transfer through the old walls and windows in this way: Instead of blowing insulation into the walls, a layer of rigid foam insulation was attached to the old exterior wall. This styrofoam comes in tongue-and-groove sheets that can be nailed. It was later covered by the brick veneer wall in the front and by the vinyl siding on the back and sides.

We had storm windows made for each of the old windows. These storm sashes, mounted on the inside frame of the old casement windows, have effectively reduced heat loss even from our waiting room's bay-window area.

The walls of the new wing of our building have both the exterior foam insulation and interior mineral wool insulation in the walls. All attic and crawl space areas have more than six inches of insulation.

There are other possibilities you may want to consider:

1. Ask your architect if solar energy is suitable for part of your building's needs. This is possible in parts of the country.

2. In some regions of the country, the availability and the price of oil changes from time to time in comparison with natural gas. Boilers are available that can be switched easily from one fuel to the other. Ask about them if you're in such an area.

3. Plants can produce major energy savings if used properly. The following appeared in the American Horticultural Society's newsletter, *News and Views*, July 1979, and is reprinted by permission. Although it's aimed at the home-owner, many of its suggestions are applicable to a small professional office building. Those that don't apply have been omitted.

"10 Ways to Conserve Energy With Plants

"**1.** Plant large deciduous shade trees on the southern, southwestern, and western sides of your [building]. Deciduous trees (which lose their leaves in winter) block the summer sun but allow full penetration of the winter's warming sun. Plant trees approximately 15 feet apart and approximately 15 feet from your [building]. Stick with the strong-wooded oaks (red, scarlet, white), lindens, or ash to avoid wind damage to buildings. Keep these orientations free of evergreen trees that will block the winter sun. A recent study showed that an 8°F difference between shaded and unshaded wall surfaces was equivalent to a 30 percent increase in insulation value for the shaded wall.

"**2.** Plant deciduous vines so they climb directly on the southern and western walls of a brick or masonry building. They block summer sun but allow the winter sun in. If your [building] is of wood, construct a trellis next to the walls of the building and encourage vine growth on the trellis. This will eliminate rotting problems created by vines on wood.

"**3.** Plant deciduous or evergreen trees and shrubs on the eastern, southern, and western sides of an outdoor air-conditioning condenser. The hotter a condenser gets, the harder it has to work. As much as a 3 percent savings in the efficiency of the air-conditioning system can be realized simply by shading the condenser from the summer's hot sun. . . .

"**4.** Plant two or more rows of evergreen trees on the north and northwest sides of your [building] to block winter winds. Windbreaks provide the greatest reduction in wind velocity at a distance of five to seven times the windbreak's height on its leeward side. Winter energy consumption has been reduced by as much as 30 percent by proper design and maintenance of windbreaks.

"**5.** Plant dense evergreen shrubs on the western, northwestern, and northern sides of your [building] to provide additional insulation against infiltration of cold-weather air into the structure. Evergreen vines on these walls (for brick structures) or near these walls (for wood buildings) will also help. . . .

"**6.** Plant trees and shrubs that will act as wind tunnels and channel the southwesterly summer breezes into and through the [building]. This may involve selective thinning of understory plants to promote maximum air circulation.

"**7.** Be sure that plant masses (groups of shrubs and/or trees) you create will allow the natural downhill flow of cooler air. This will promote more circulation in the summer and avoid creating "cold air lakes" near your [building] in the winter.

"**8.** In selecting colors for plant and construction materials, stick with medium to darker tones. Darker colors are more efficient absorbers of the winter sun's warmth. As long as darker-colored materials are properly shaded by deciduous shade trees, their heat retaining qualities can be moderated in the summer.

"**9.** Where feasible, deflect air from exhaust vents, air conditioners, etc. out of areas with plantings. Preferably, these sources of hot air should be exhausted into northern orientations where heat excesses are not as severe."

27
CONTROLLING POLLUTION IN THE OFFICE ENVIRONMENT

Some office pollution is hazardous, some merely annoying. For the safety and contentment of everyone who comes to your office, you have to keep both kinds under control.

RADIATION

If your office will have any kind of X-ray equipment, you and your architect will have to consider the need for radiation shielding.

During the 1970s many states enacted increasingly stringent laws to protect the patient, the doctor, and the staff from hazardous radiation. New York, for example, requires periodic recalibration and recertification of all X-ray equipment. All new installations must have lead-lined walls and, in some cases, doors, ceilings, and floors.

If your suite needs this sort of radiation protection, your architect should get a copy of the lead-shielding requirements. The equipment supplier may be able to provide this, but to be certain you have the most up-to-date rules, you should get them directly from the state agency involved.

New York has a list of licensed radiation physicists who act as inspectors. We called in one of them while our plans were still in the preliminary stage. On a copy of our floor plan, we marked the proposed location of our present and future X-ray equipment. He then marked which walls required lead lining, the thickness of lead needed, where it was to be installed, and where the equipment operator must stand during an exposure. Several months later, when the walls were framed, and the exact location of each piece of X-ray equipment had been decided on, the inspector returned and marked for the builder the exact parts of each involved wall that needed shielding. We then knew we were in compliance with the code, and we kept the use of expensive shielding to a minimum.

There are several ways to install the lead. Probably the best and least expensive is the purchase of sheets of leaded wallboard. The required thickness of lead comes glued to the back surface of the wallboard, so both are nailed to the wall together. For the shielding to be complete, all electrical outlet boxes must also be wrapped with lead.

AIR POLLUTION

The air in a dental or medical suite can easily become unpleasant or unhealthy or both. As you plan for your new office, you can prepare to prevent or control the major forms of interior pollution:

1. Stale air can be exchanged for fresh by having windows that open, by having an air-conditioning system that introduces outside air, and by the use of exhaust fans.

2. Unpleasant odors can be prevented by prompt disposal of soiled or bloody materials (see section below on garbage handling) and by thorough cleaning of equipment such as aspirator nozzles and hoses. While odor-masking substances are sometimes used in lavatories, prompt air turnover with an exhaust fan ducted to the outside is more effective.

3. Smoke has no place in a doctor's office. Smoking should be prohibited.

4. Nitrous-oxide contamination of the office air can be reduced to a negligible level by proper ventilation and by the use of a scavenging nose mask by the patient.

NOISE POLLUTION

The control of sound in the medical or dental office involves two broad concerns: the elimination or muting of unwanted noises originating inside or outside the office, and the protection of the confidentiality of conversations with and about patients relating to health, finances, and other personal matters.

Before we discuss specific techniques for controlling sound, let's review how sound behaves. Sound leaves its source as continually enlarging spheres, a three-dimensional series of ripples that diminish in intensity with distance. When sound hits a surface, part of its energy is transmitted, part is absorbed—depending on the character of the surface—and part is blocked or reflected. The way to reduce sound pollution is to *keep unwanted sound at a distance*, *prevent its transmission*, or *absorb it*. If any or all of these are ineffective, you can try to *mask* it. Let's consider each of these approaches.

Distance. Whenever possible, keep noise-producing equipment out of the office. A basement is the best location for a compressor or a central suction pump. If this solution is impossible, these items should be placed in the most remote portion of the office, such as between the lab and an outside wall. If such a location simply can't be arranged, you may have to resort to some of the other measures discussed below.

The proper zoning of your office floor plan will also apply the distance solution to other sounds. The farther your waiting room is from the treatment rooms, for example, the less audible to the waiting patients will be such anxiety-producing noises as the crying of a frightened child patient or the whine of some piece of equipment. Similarly, if your consultation room/private office is far from the waiting room, it may need less acoustical treatment of walls, ceiling, and floor.

Obviously, distance is most practical for the muting of sounds in the fairly large office, but even in a small suite, proper planning will help. One means of reducing sound transmission across hallways, for example, is to stagger the placement of the doors so that no doorway is directly opposite that of the room across the hall.

Blocking the sound (transmission prevention). Sound is transmitted freely through the air, but to a lesser extent through solid materials. The denser and thicker the material, the more sound transmission is blocked. A cinderblock wall allows less sound to pass through than does an ordinary Sheetrock partition. Similarly, a double thickness of wallboard blocks sound far better than does a single layer. Openings in walls, ceilings, or floors reduce the sound-limiting effects of all solid materials.

Absorbing the sound. Certain materials admit sound and then trap it in a series of small chambers. The sound reverberates within these chambers until its energy is dissipated. These materials include soft substances, such as carpeting, drapes, and fibrous insulation, as well as firm acoustic ceiling panels and rigid plastic foams. Acoustic engineers evaluate the sound-absorbing quality of a substance in terms of its noise reduction coefficient. The higher the NRC—to a theoretical maximum of 1.00—the more it deadens sound.

Masking. The use of pleasant sounds to hide unpleasant sounds is sometimes called "acoustic perfume." Its most common application in the business office is the use of background music. These systems are discussed in Chapter 32. The ring of a telephone is a kind of sound pollution if it occurs frequently throughout the day. We found that replacing the bell with a pleasant chime makes it much more tolerable. *White noise*, a mixture of sound produced by a special generator, is sometimes used to mask a high ambient noise level in large business offices.

Now let's apply these four principles of sound control to different components of the office:

Ceilings. The acoustic panels forming a dropped ceiling are usually suspended from the structural ceiling, such as the slab of the floor above in a high-rise office building, by metal wires or straps. The panels are made of a porous mineral substance that usually has a high NRC—at least 0.75.

This means that your ceiling would absorb 75 percent of the sound striking it *if* the ceiling contained nothing but the acoustic material. It doesn't. It also usually has light fixtures, air-conditioning registers, loudspeaker baffles, and sometimes an exposed portion of the ceiling-supporting metal framework. All of these hard surfaces reflect sound back into the room and can conduct it to other rooms. In addition, there are air gaps at corners, near walls, and between the panels where they rest on the framework. These gaps can transmit sound unless they're plugged with caulking or the top of the dropped ceiling is covered by more sound absorbing material, such as batts of insulation.

Sound transmission from room to room through ventilating ducts above the ceiling can be reduced by having the interior of the ducts insulated; this is often desirable for energy conservation and to avoid condensation as well. Bends or baffles in the ducts also reduce sound passage.

Be sure that the ceiling material you choose complies with local fire regulations and that its support system doesn't violate the building code, as did the system installed for a doctor friend of mine who was his own general contractor. His ceiling grid had to be completely removed and a new one installed.

Acoustic ceilings come in many different surface textures and patterns. While you will seldom look directly at your ceiling, your patients will, as they lie on an examining table or recline in a dental chair. Pick a pattern and a texture that are restful to look at. A concealed suspension ceiling (a *spline* ceiling) is the most effective soundproofing, but it's also the most expensive.

Floors. The sound-absorbing property of carpeting is second only to that of acoustic ceiling materials. The NRC for carpeting ranges up to 0.55, regardless of the material used. It can be in the upper range if a heavier weight pile and/or a higher pile are used. The sound-absorbing property can be increased up to NRC 0.65 to 0.70 by the use of padding under the carpet. In contrast, sheet vinyl, vinyl asbestos tile, or other resilient floor coverings have an NRC of only about 0.05.

Thus, it makes sense from the standpoint of acoustics to carpet most of the floors. We'll discuss in Chapter 39 how to select carpeting and when it would be better not to use it.

Walls. Your walls can be built to block sound transmission and/or to absorb any sound energy that passes through the outer surface. Figure 27-1 shows some of the methods used.

You and your architect may decide to use one or a combination of these methods, depending on the likely severity of the problem.

Doors. A solid-core door is superior to one with a hollow core, as far as soundproofing is concerned. But for more complete blockage of sound, it's necessary to install weather-stripping around the edges of the door to prevent as much air passage as possible.

Total control of sound passage through doors is generally possible only with a double-door arrangement. A second door is installed a few feet behind the

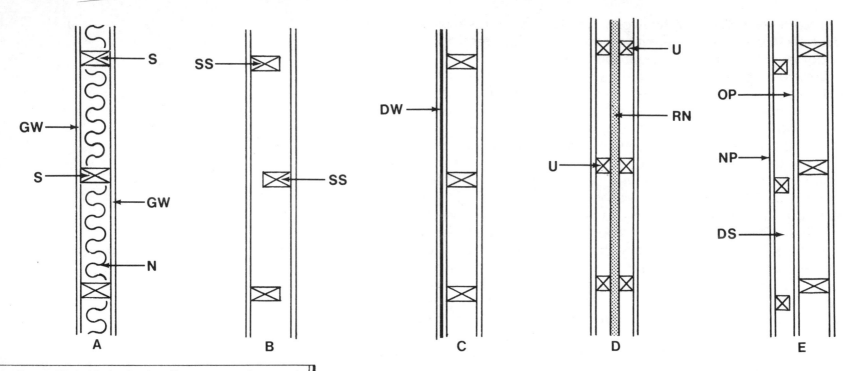

Figure 27-1. Methods of wall construction for sound control. **A:** Standard interior partition has two-by-four stud centers (S) 16 inches apart, with gypsum wallboard (GW) nailed to each side. Empty space in wall may be filled with batts of mineral insulation (N) to absorb sound. **B:** Staggered studs (SS) are arranged so that no stud contacts both sides of wall, thereby minimizing sound conduction. **C:** Double layer of wallboard (DW) on one side of wall helps to block sound transmission. **D:** Wall is built with two-by-twos (U) instead of two-by-fours, with one-inch-thick, rigid, sound absorbing insulation (RN) in center. **E:** New partition (NP) is built with two-by-fours in front of and not touching an existing wall (OP), leaving dead space (DS) between them. Sometimes combinations of these methods are used, such as filling wall in B, C, or E with batts of insulation.

first, and both of them are weather-stripped. This arrangement is seen most often in psychiatrists' offices.

Windows are likely to be a problem in noise control if your office building is located on a busy street. Distance from the noise helps; offices on upper floors in a high-rise building will be much less affected.

To reduce sound transmission through the windows, insulated (two-layer) glass is helpful. Sometimes, a third sheet of glass is installed inside the window frame. If the noise level is still too high, you may have to hang heavy drapes over the windows. Since this will block out light as well as sound, it should be considered only as a last resort. Other possibilities include construction of a fence between the building and the street and the planting of trees to serve as an acoustic barrier.

Equipment such as compressors or central suction pumps sometimes must be placed in closets or other locations within the office. If you expect to have this problem, there are measures you can take to muffle the noise level:

1. Select equipment that is relatively quiet. This immediately prevents part of the noise problem. If necessary, go to the dealer's showroom and listen to several different models in operation.

2. Provide sound barriers and insulation. If the equipment is to be in a closet, line the walls and ceiling of the closet with acoustic ceiling tile. Use a solid-core door and have it weather-stripped. Note that this may cause overheating of the motor if the closet is a small one with no source of outside air. Find out from the dealer or the equipment manufacturer how much air supply is needed. You may need a vent with acoustic baffles. Plan for this in your *original* construction, not later.

3. If the equipment must be in the corner of a room that cannot be closed off as can a closet, have your carpenter make a plywood enclosure lined with acoustic ceiling tile or other sound-absorptive material. Again, be careful about providing adequate air to the equipment.

4. Isolate the equipment from the floor. The frame should rest on some type of cushioning material, such as rubber feet or a foam pad. This will minimize transmission of the vibration to the rest of the office.

VISUAL POLLUTION

Think about the visual aspects of your office from two viewpoints: First, how to present those things that are to be seen; this category refers to decorating the office and is discussed in Part VII. Second, how to keep out of sight those things that you don't want seen; in other words, control of visual pollution. Think about these possibilities:

1. Arrange treatment rooms so that a patient being examined does not feel exposed to the view of those in the hallway if someone should open the door.

2. Keep soiled or bloody instruments out of sight prior to cleaning and sterilizing. This can be done by covering or wrapping them, or by soaking them in a deep sink.

3. Arrange a staff lounge area out of sight of patients. Your assistant may be entitled to her mid-morning cup of coffee, but if she drinks it in view of patients she'll look as if she's not working, or she'll be thought rude for not offering coffee to the watching patients.

4. Cover with blinds or curtains those windows that have unappealing views.

5. Reduce the closed-in feeling of interior rooms by the use of wall murals depicting outdoor scenes.

6. Be certain that cleanliness and neatness are maintained all through the working day, especially in the waiting room and the patients' lavatory. One of your assistant's regular duties should be rearranging disordered magazines and picking up litter.

7. Have trash containers that are adequate in size and are emptied frequently. The sight of overflowing trash baskets may diminish patients' respect for the doctor and the staff.

GARBAGE DISPOSAL

The increasing use of disposables has made the trash-control problem a significant one in many professional offices. Every room where disposables are used should have an adequate waste receptacle.

We found that the best type holds at least half a day's—or better, a full day's—waste, has a wide mouth to minimize missed throws, is deep enough so that patients won't see its contents, and has a mouth that is open all the time rather than one that requires stepping on a pedal or pushing a swinging door.

You'll need different-sized cans, depending on the amount of anticipated waste. We found that the ideal container for three of our rooms is the one shown in Figure 42-1, which meets the requirements mentioned above. It comes with a swinging door that we removed. Since its opening is on the side instead of the center of the top, we can keep it under the countertop, out of the way but accessible.

You're likely to find a wider variety of receptacles in the catalogs of commercial office or industrial-supply companies than in those of medical or dental suppliers. If you decide to keep the can under a counter, be sure you know before ordering it how much clearance you'll have between the floor and the underside of the counter. In other words, decide on the counter height before ordering the can. (Cabinets and countertops are discussed in Chapter 42.)

Make special provision for disposal of hazardous substances, such as used needles, chemicals, and contaminated articles.

Once the trash has been collected, what will you do with it? If, in your locality, garbage is picked up nightly, you'll need only a location where one or several large cans or plastic bags can be left.

Our office is in a suburban village in which garbage is collected only once a week. To avoid having many unsightly garbage cans near our side entrance, we bought a trash compactor, which we keep in the staff room. This compresses an entire week's garbage to fit into one 32-gallon can. Since the filled can is often heavy, we bought one with wheels mounted on it for rolling it to the curb on pickup day.

Consider the use of a compactor, also, if your office is so small that even one or two days' accumulated waste will be in the way. Plan for it in terms of location. They are usually 34 inches high, made to fit under kitchen counters. You'll need a 110-volt outlet nearby.

28
TELEPHONES: SHOULD YOU RENT OR SHOULD YOU BUY?

The telephone is one piece of equipment that is found in the office of every doctor. Depending on your type of practice, your phone bill may range from $600 to $6,000 or more per year.

Until the past few years, you had no choice when obtaining your phone. The local phone company was the only source and it *rented* the equipment to you. With recent court decisions, another source became available. You can now *buy* your equipment outright.

Should you consider buying? The answer is a tentative Yes, but before we discuss the costs, benefits, and problems of owning your own telephone equipment, it's worthwhile to look at your present phone bill.

There's a fixed amount listed on your bill that you must pay even if you make no calls during the month. The charges for calls, federal tax, and local tax (if any) are added to the fixed amount to arrive at the monthly total.

The fixed amount is itself made up of several parts: The *equipment charge* is based on the number and complexity of the phones in your office—the number of telephones, hold buttons, line buttons, volume controls, intercoms, buzzers, and other options.

This chapter first appeared in slightly altered form in *Dental Management*, February 1979. It is reprinted by permission from *Dental Management*. Copyright © 1979 Harcourt Brace Jovanovich Inc.

The *line charge* is based on how many central office lines (phone numbers) you have and whether your phones have Touch Tone instead of a dial.

Other fixed charges may be added for such items as directory listings or a mileage charge if you have an answering service.

The equipment charge is the only portion of your phone bill that can be reduced by buying your phones, but this reduction can be substantial, especially if you plan to have many phone instruments in your office.

Two types of companies exist now, which were largely unknown a few years ago: The *telephone broker*, or *communications consultant*, is essentially a salesman who'll discuss your phone needs with you, plan your system, and then return later with a formal proposal. This is a written list of the equipment you'll need and the costs involved. He'll get these figures from the one or more *interconnect companies* with which he works. The salesman earns a commission on the sale of the equipment. He may oversee the equipment installation, but he doesn't do the work himself. He may also negotiate with the local telephone company on your behalf in arranging for the installation.

An *interconnect company* provides the telephone instruments and installs the wiring in your office. It's also responsible for the servicing and maintenance of the instruments. Typically, replacement parts and service are provided without charge for a year. Thereafter, you can buy a service contract if you wish.

How much can you save by buying your phones? It's difficult to answer that question, because there are many different elements involved, but let's try to sort them out.

Table 28-1 is an example of a 10-year cost projection of three different ways to obtain phone service. Two of them are available from the phone company. The third is a purchased system. In each case, the 1980 base prices were obtained from companies involved. The projections are my own calculations based on what I believe to be reasonable assumptions.

Each system is a Touch Tone, nine-telephone arrangement with three phone numbers and a dial intercom.

The standard key sets (first column) are the traditional six-button models (five line buttons plus a hold button) that have been in use for 20 years or more. The pricing of the special key sets (second column) is an attempt by the phone

TABLE 28-1

Rented Versus Purchased Telephone Systems
10-Year Cost Projection

	Phone company standard key sets	Phone company special key sets	Purchased interconnect system
Equipment cost	$18,366[1]	"A" rate: $ 5,530[2] "B" rate: 6,768[3]	$4,000
Rate increases—cumulative at 10% per year[4]	10,905	"B" rate: 4,018	None
Local taxes 4% (varies by locality)	1,171	653	160
Installation	1,145	114	125
Maintenance	None	None	2,869[5]
Subtotal	$31,587	$17,083	$7,154
Investment tax credit	None	None	−400
Total cost	$31,587	$17,083	$6,754

Notes for Table 28-1

(1) Amount shown is $153 per month (1980 rate), projected over 10 years. Subject to rate increases.

(2) "A" rate is one-time charge for this system. Can be paid as lump sum or over three, five, or seven years, with carrying charges added. Not subject to charge over 10 years. Subject to rate increases.

(3) "B" rate is a monthly charge for this system ($56.40 per month in 1980). Amount shown is this charge projected over 10 years. Subject to rate increases.

(4) Based on past history of increases in rates for business-telephone equipment.

(5) Assumes 1980 cost of maintenance (parts and labor) contract as $20 per phone per year ($180 per year for this system), with cumulative annual increases of 10 percent per year. Such a contract is not mandatory. Service may be paid for, instead, on a per-visit basis.

company to compete with the private interconnect systems. They bring down the cost substantially in comparison with the standard key sets, but their cost is still well above that of private systems.

My projection, of necessity, is oversimplified. The net after-tax cost has not been calculated. Payments to the phone company are deductible in the year you pay them, but a purchased system is depreciated over a number of years. Also, telephone company rented systems are replaced immediately without charge if they are lost in a fire or flood, while private systems must be insured. In addition, the costs of updating each system with new technological features couldn't be included. I've omitted interest costs because I'm assuming that lump sums are paid for either the private system or the telephone company's "A" rate.

Before you make a decision on your own phone system, do your own complete analysis or ask your accountant to do it. Don't rely on a cost projection provided by either the phone company or an interconnect company. Each is likely to be biased.

What's the catch? If the numbers in Table 28-1 are even close to being correct, why doesn't everyone rush out to buy equipment? These and other questions are reasonable and must be considered

In many parts of the country, more doctors, other professionals, and businesses are buying their telephone equipment than ever before, but many are not. Why? These are some of the reasons:

1. The chief concern is service. If your rented phones don't work, the phone company's repair crew will usually be there within a few hours. You can be confident that the phone company will still be in business one or 10 years from now. Interconnect companies, on the other hand, are a recent development. Most of them are small businesses and, as in any new field, a certain percentage of them will be incompetent and/or unscrupulous. If the company you deal with goes out of business, you may lose all or part of your deposit if the bankruptcy occurs before the installation is completed. If the business fails later on, you may lose any amount you've paid toward a service contract. In addition, you'll have to find another interconnect company to service your phones. We'll suggest ways to minimize these risks later in this chapter.

2. The office is temporary. If the new location is not one you expect to occupy for many years, it will often be less expensive to rent your phones. Of course, you can take purchased phones with you when you move, since they are your property, but the colors may not be correct for another office, and you might want a different combination of wall and desk units in another new location.

3. The telephone company's local lines have frequent problems. I know of at least one community where cross talk between lines, static, and low sound volume are common. A local law firm decided not to buy their phones because it could be difficult to distinguish problems within a purchased system from those on the phone company's lines. They were afraid that the phone company and the interconnect company each would blame the other's equipment, while they were left stranded with inoperative phones. Problems of this sort can be at least partly overcome by a method discussed below.

4. Inertia. Many established offices rent phones because they have always done so, and they continue to rent them when they move.

If you want to take advantage of the substantial savings often involved in a purchased phone system, how can you protect yourself from the hazards just mentioned? Here is a reasonable sequence to follow:

1. Decide on your telephone needs—the number of lines, number of instruments, dial or Touch Tone, intercom, and other special features, such as hands-off capability, volume controls, or call diverters. Don't forget to include possible future expansion.

2. Obtain quotations for the system from several interconnect companies and from the phone company. Be sure all costs are included and labeled. For example, ask the interconnect company if maintenance charges are being lumped together with the purchase price. This might happen if the quotation is for an installment purchase. Ask to have them separated.

Ask the telephone company about *termination charges* for the system. This is an amount levied if the special key sets are removed from your office within a specified period after installment. It could be significant if you decide later to go to a purchased system.

Get all the figures from the phone company and from each interconnect company for federal, state, and local taxes, installation, shipping, "cut-over" charges (connection of a purchased system to phone company lines), maintenance (on a service contract and a per-visit basis), insurance (for a private system), and interest (for installment purchases).

3. Work out your own cost comparison with your accountant's help on the tax aspects. The basic question to answer is whether the savings to be expected are enough to make such an investment worthwhile. Some analysts have noted that a purchased phone system is cost-effective if your office needs at least five telephones on three lines. But you should calculate the costs for yourself before you decide.

4. If purchase of a system seems reasonable, select one or two interconnect companies that are highly recommended.

The question of service calls must be considered first because even one day without a working phone system can result in the loss of appreciable income due to missed appointments. This is why you must do some careful checking of the interconnect company.

Ask them how long they've been in business at their present or past address. Have they ever operated under another name? Ask for a list of customers to whom they've sold phones, especially systems with the same features you're seeking. How long ago was the first one installed? Call these references and ask about the service provided. This track record is very important. If it's too short or if some of the customers have reservations about the firm, be wary!

A second precaution is to have your local credit bureau investigate the company. The credit bureau will turn up any liens on judgments against the company by dissatisfied customers. These will be customers whose names the company did not give to you. I would try to speak to those customers also, as well as to the Better Business Bureau.

If the reports you get about the company or companies in your area give you cause for concern, *stay away!* Stick with the phone company. You can be certain that it will be in business and able to service your phones.

On the other hand, if the interconnect company has been in business for several years, if you have spoken to a substantial number of satisfied customers, and if there are few or no liens or judgments against the company, it should be safe to proceed.

5. Have your attorney review the contract with the interconnect company before you sign it. The contract will probably include your authorization for the interconnect company to negotiate on your behalf with the phone company for the installation. For a complete discussion of interconnect systems, including items to be included in the contract, see Roger J. St. Onge's article "Interconnect—The New Alternative" in *Medical Group Management*, March/April 1979.

6. Plan for placement of the junction box where the phone company's lines and the interconnect company's wiring are joined. This should be in your basement or utility room. An electrical outlet must be available nearby, and this line must always be hot—that is, not on your master electrical shut-off. And don't forget to order a jack for your answering machine if you plan to use one.

7. Here's how to find out whether troubles with a system are in your purchased equipment or in the phone company's lines. In the northeast, and probably elsewhere, for each central office line (phone number) you are entitled to one black single-line telephone from the phone company, without extra cost, even if your system is purchased. Thus, if you have three lines you can get three black phones, either wall or desk models.

The neatest arrangement is to have the phone company install a jack near your secretary's desk for each line. Order the black phones as plug-in desk models. Keep them stored in a closet out of the way. They are a form of insurance, which works as follows: Suppose that one day your purchased phones don't work. Your secretary then plugs in one of the black phones and tries to make a call. If the black phone works properly on incoming and outgoing calls while your private system does not, the problem is in your own system. Call the interconnect company for service. Until the repair is made, your secretary can use one or all of the black phones for normal office needs.

If neither your own phones nor the black phones work properly, the problem is likely to be somewhere in the phone company's equipment. Send someone out to another phone to call the repair department.

This kind of diagnosis is valuable in another way. If you call for the phone company's repair service and the problem turns out to be in your private equipment, you'll be charged at least $25 or $30 by the phone company for the service call, although they won't repair your private equipment. You'll still have to call the interconnect company to make the repair. You'll save time and money by tracking down the malfunction.

8. If you'll need new phone numbers, be sure to reserve them with the phone company well in advance, so you'll have plenty of time to order announcements and new stationery, and so that the number or numbers will be in the next edition of the phone directory, if the timing is right.

One final thought: If the interconnect company goes out of business and your office is in a large metropolitan area, you'll probably be able to find another company to service your equipment. A way to lessen your exposure to serious servicing problems is to buy phone equipment that is widely used. Well-known American-made equipment can be maintained by almost any interconnect company. Little-known equipment, on the other hand, especially if foreign-made, may use different circuitry and may require special parts and training for maintenance. If you buy this type and the interconnect company fails, you may have a more difficult problem finding another company to take over the servicing.

What did we do? We bought our telephone equipment in 1978. After some minor initial problems, it's worked well for us, and the savings have been as expected.

PLANNING YOUR PHONE LOCATIONS

You can avoid a constant, needless source of annoyance to your secretary by giving some thought to the placement of her phone. You'll want her to be able to dial easily and to use the phone without having its coiled wire draped across the appointment book.

Order a desk phone with a cable that comes out of the wall next to her desk just above desk height, not down near the floor. Be sure the cable from the wall to the phone is long enough to permit placement of the phone anywhere on the desk. With the telephone at her left and the receiver in her left hand, your right-handed secretary can write with the desk top in front of her unencumbered by trailing wires. Reverse the phone placement for a left-hander. If she'll ever have to move away from her desk while on the phone, order a long coiled cord for her instrument.

The same kind of thinking should enable you to plan the location of your private-office phone. We find that a wall phone is efficient here and avoids one more item on the desk (see Figure 41-5).

If you plan to have wall phones in treatment rooms above cabinets, have them positioned high enough so that the coiled wire doesn't interfere with use of the countertop (see Figure 42-1).

Mark the location of each phone on your floor plan with the height above the floor at which the wires should exit from the wall.

29
SIGNALING SYSTEMS AND INTERCOMS

The use of devices for communicating within the office arises from these basic concerns:

1. The need to deliver messages from one part of the office to another without walking from room to room. Increases in numbers of rooms and staff members make this need more compelling.

2. The desirability of delivering some messages without patients being aware of them.

Based on my own informal survey of doctors, the most commonly needed messages are to:

☐ summon an assistant to a particular room;

☐ inform doctor or assistant that the next patient has arrived;

☐ inform doctor of a phone call with or without specifying its nature;

☐ inform doctor that a patient being prepared by an assistant is now ready for doctor;

☐ tell secretary or another staff member to pick up phone for instructions;

☐ tell secretary or assistant that doctor is ready for next patient; and

☐ inform doctor and/or staff that a particular room is empty or occupied.

Note that except for calling an assistant to a particular room, some degree of privacy from patients is desirable for virtually all of the messages. This means that unless the system used can offer this privacy, it needs improvement.

On the list above, mark those messages that are likely to be used in your office and add any special ones of your own. Once you've done this, you'll be able to plan your own system.

The perfect system doesn't exist, but if it did I'd want it to have these qualities:

1. It would deliver the message accurately, completely, and only to the intended recipient, who could respond to it completely.

2. It would be simple, inexpensive, and easy to install and maintain.

3. It would require minimal effort to initiate a message and to respond. It would not require touching anything with a scrubbed or gloved hand.

4. Neither the message nor the response would disturb others working in the office or be discerned by patients.

Table 29-1 lists some of the possible systems you can consider. After reading it, think about these ideas:

TABLE 29-1

Systems for Communications Within the Office

Method	Advantages	Disadvantages
Speaking face to face	Messages are accurate, immediate, complete, and go only to intended recipient. Response is immediate and complete. Unnecessary for doctor to touch anything.	Requires walking room to room. Not private if patient is present.
Face to face using hand or other signals	Messages go only to intended recipient. Response is immediate. Patient is unaware of meaning. Doctor does not have to touch anything.	Requires walking room to room. Only a limited number of messages and responses possible. Complicated message may be misunderstood. Response usually limited to a nod by doctor.
Audible signal only (buzzer, tone, bell)	Simple and inexpensive to install and maintain. Patients hear signal but are unaware of meaning.	Messages severely limited in number and complexity. Doctor must touch button to reply.
Intercom, using telephone handset (it may be part of the phone system or a separate intercom)	Messages and responses are accurate, immediate, and complete. If system has dial feature, messages go only to intended recipient.	Doctor must pick up handset (and then wash hands). Patient hears half of conversation.

If you're planning to use some form of voice intercom, your first decision should be whether to incorporate it in your office telephone system or to buy separate intercom equipment.

1. Include it in your phone system only if you buy rather than rent your phones. If you buy your telephones, the voice intercom feature is easily added for a small extra cost, since it uses the same instruments and the same wiring as the phones. If you'll have rooms that need intercoms, but not regular telephones, you can buy an intercom unit for those rooms.

2. Buy a separate complete intercom system if you use phone company telephones. This advice is based on the phone company's high monthly rental

Method	Advantages	Disadvantages
Intercom with hands-off feature (part of phone system or separate)	Messages and responses are accurate, immediate, and complete. Unnecessary for doctor to touch anything (no handwashing). Can be combined with a handset intercom.	Not private when hands-off feature used. Like a public-address system unless it has dial feature to direct call to a specific room.
Visible (silent): Series of lights that can be turned on in different combinations; lights remain on until reset button is pressed; audible signal calls attention to lights	Large number of possible messages. Inconspicuous. Lights continue to deliver message after audible signal ends. Patients unaware of meaning. Code can direct message to specific individual. Units are attractive, blend with decor. Defective unit can be bypassed so rest of system can operate. May be combined with voice intercom.	Expensive: Most cost well over $200 per room, including wiring. Wireless units cost more. Defective unit requires call for serviceman or sending unit back to manufacturer. Since person sending message may not know location of intended recipient, lights go on and tone sounds throughout office. Everyone must look up from work. Recipient must respond promptly, otherwise system cannot be used for other messages. Must be used for simple, frequently needed messages only. Attempts to transmit complicated messages lead to errors or nonuse. Requires doctor to press button.

charges for extra equipment added to their phones. For example, the phone company will rent to you for about $1.17 per phone per month (1980) a simple signal buzzer that alerts you to pick up the phone for an intercom message. Yet each buzzer costs perhaps $5 or less. Thus for each phone, you'll be paying more than *double* the total cost of that buzzer *each year*. Multiply that by the number of phones, add the comparable rental charges for other equipment needed to operate the intercom, and you'll see why it doesn't pay to rent an intercom from the phone company.

3. If you buy a separate voice intercom system, have the wiring installed while the walls are open. Before you do that, though, think about whether you want a silent system—light signals—as well. If you do, now is the time to plan for it and to have the necessary wiring installed during construction.

Notice that I've been speaking only of *wired* units. If you install an intercom system while the office is being built or renovated, that's probably the best type to use, since the wires can easily be hidden inside the walls. But if you need an intercom later, you might consider a wireless system either with just voice communication or voice plus a panel of lights.

These wireless units usually operate by superimposing an electronic signal on the office's 110-volt AC lines. They are sometimes called "carrier current" systems. Each station is hung on the wall and plugged into a nearby outlet.

Such systems have their own merits and drawbacks. On the plus side, they can be delivered and operated immediately, with no waiting for installation. There is no interruption of office procedures while holes are drilled and cables are snaked through the walls and over a dropped ceiling. Expansion of the system at a later date involves only buying additional stations and plugging them in. If you move, the entire system goes with you by just unplugging the units.

But there are disadvantages, too. Because of their more complicated electronic circuitry, wireless systems cost substantially more than wired ones with the same capabilities. In some cases, the price differential exceeds the added labor costs involved in wired systems. More serious is the possibility of electrical interference in your building. If there is some defective electrical or electronic equipment nearby, the background hum or crackling in the wireless system could prove to be objectionable. For this reason, if I were considering using a wireless intercom system, I'd want to use it in my own office for a period of time on approval.

With any type of intercom, voice or silent, there are other points to consider:

1. In the simplest voice systems, a call initiated at one station can be heard at all other stations. If you want to direct calls to only one specific station, you'll need a *dial intercom,* or some other way of informing a particular person that the message is just for her or him.

2. Will you want a unit outside your office's entry door to find out who's there before admitting them? Many offices in big-city buildings are now using these for security.

3. If you choose a hands-off voice system, get a handset for each station, too, for confidential messages.

4. If you are going to buy an expensive system for a rented office, have a clause inserted in your lease, entitling you to take the system with you when you move. Otherwise, the landlord can claim that because they're installed in the walls the units are his property.

5. Keep it simple! This is especially important for systems of lights. Complex combinations of lights for infrequently used messages lead to errors and diminished use. Elaborate systems are more expensive to buy, install, and repair.

6. Can the system be repaired by local service people or by you? Other things being equal, a local company will provide prompter service than a distant one, but if a system ordered by mail is made up of easily replaceable modules you can probably service it yourself by disconnecting the defective unit or parts and sending them back for repair or replacement.

7. A single defective station shouldn't put the entire system out of operation. The company should provide a troubleshooting manual.

8. The system you buy should be expandable; you may enlarge the office and need more stations.

9. Find out the track record of the system by calling other doctors who are using it. Ask about the system's reliability, usefulness, need for service, ease of service, and general user satisfaction.

10. If you're considering a silent system, find out if the lights that deliver the messages can be separated from the buttons you'll press to initiate or to respond to a message. The best place for the lights is on the wall opposite your usual working position in each room, but the most convenient spot for the buttons is close to you, on or just under a countertop, attached to a mobile cabinet, an examining table, or a dental chair.

11. If several doctors work in the office at the same time, the system should permit directing voice or silent messages to one without disturbing the others.

12. Some of the more elaborate systems offer options you might find useful. For example, a few can include a background music system with speakers in each room.

13. Some wired systems have prewired connectors at both ends of each cable. These are plugged into the back of the unit. Other systems use color-coded wires with bared ends that are screwed to terminals on the back of the unit. Each manufacturer claims that his method is best, but each has its own advantages and disadvantages. Prewired connectors are easy to plug in when a unit is installed or removed for servicing, since each wire doesn't have to be individually stripped and then attached. But prewired connectors also make it necessary to buy precut lengths of cable with the connectors attached—you're forced to buy more cable than the length you need—and the size of the connector may make it necessary to drill larger holes in walls and ceiling than would be needed without the connectors.

We decided on the following communications systems for our own office:

Voice intercom. This is an integral part of the telephone system we bought. Each of the four treatment rooms now used by the doctors has a telephone, as does each doctor's desk, the receptionist, the insurance clerk, and the bookkeeper. The intercom is a dial type: A message for a particular person can be directed to that person's station by the caller (the term dial-intercom is used even though the phone has buttons instead of a dial).

Each doctor is likely to be in one of three rooms at most times during the day. The system is arranged so that to reach me, for example, the receptionist presses 9. This causes the phone to buzz at my desk and in each of the two treatment rooms which I use.

Assistant call system. To summon an assistant, we press a button, either at a doctor's desk or in a treatment room, which causes a tone to sound momentarily in a central location (the sterilizing alcove). At the same time, a light goes on in the hall just outside the room where the assistant is needed. The bright green light stays on until the assistant presses a reset button under the light.

I designed, built, and installed this arrangement myself, since I was unable to find one ready for purchase at the time we needed it. (See Chapter 61). It's likely, however, that such a system could be supplied by one of the companies that make nurse call signals for hospitals.

A variation of such a system is one with colored lights outside each treatment room to inform staff members of the status of the room—unoccupied, patient waiting, doctor with patient. Physicians should find such a system useful. Some of the companies listed below sell these systems.

We have not yet found a need in our practice for one of the multilight silent systems, but many of my doctor friends are using them and are happy with them.

Listed below are nationwide companies that sell visible (silent) intercoms. Some sell through equipment dealers only, whereas others will deal with you directly. Inclusion on the list does not imply a recommendation. You'll have to do your own investigating. There are so many companies selling voice intercoms that I haven't attempted to list them here. If you're going to buy a voice intercom that is to be separate from your telephone system, use your Yellow Pages or friends for the names of local installers.

Wired Systems

Theta Corporation
P.O. Box 806
Niagara Falls, N.Y. 14302

Monday Industries
P.O. Box 266
Westwood, N.J. 07675

A.E. Electronics Corp. (Visicom)
111 West 27th Street
New York, N.Y. 10001

Chemetron Corporation (Sicom)
696 Hampshire Road
P.O. Box 5001
Westlake Village, Calif. 91359

Signacom Systems Inc.
303 Convention Way (Suite 5)
Redwood City, Calif. 94063

Porter Instrument Co. Inc.
P.O. Box 326
Township Line Road
Hatfield, Pa. 19440

Simplified Systems Inc.
(The Communicators)
940 Lincoln Road (Suite 217)
Miami Beach, Fla. 33139

Wireless Systems

Camtek Inc.
1337 Pearl Street
Waukesha, Wis. 53186

30
ACCIDENT PREVENTION

The need for a safe office is obvious, but less obvious are the means for making your workplace hazard-free for patients, staff, and yourself. Some measures for controlling pollution have been discussed in Chapter 27. Other aspects of office safety which should be considered in your office planning are discussed here.

Preventing collisions, slips, and falls:
☐ Avoid highly polished floor surfaces and loose floor mats.
☐ Provide a stepladder—not a chair—for reaching high places.
☐ Have enough electrical outlets to avoid the use of extension cords.
☐ Keep furniture and equipment out of halls and passages.
☐ Plan wide hallways, especially at corners and at places where people may congregate.

Preventing injury from hitting or being hit by objects:
☐ Attach file cabinets, especially lateral files, to the wall. While most such cabinets have interlocks that are supposed to prevent more than one drawer from opening at a time, occasionally this interlock is bypassed, accidentally or deliberately. With two drawers open simultaneously, the cabinet can tip forward, causing serious injury and the scattering of hundreds of charts.
☐ Avoid doors that open into a hallway or other heavily traveled area.
☐ Illuminate storage and utility areas adequately.
☐ Make certain that clear glass doors and glass panels at your secretary's desk are easily recognizable.
☐ Avoid table lamps that can tip easily, especially if children will be in your waiting room.
☐ Have countertops and exposed shelves made with rounded corners.

Preventing chemical hazards:

☐ Spills are likely if tanks filled with X-ray developer and fixer must be carried far from the darkroom for cleaning. A darkroom sink of adequate size will prevent this.

☐ Acids and other caustic materials must be stored in suitable containers and in locations where breaking or spilling is unlikely.

31
OFFICE SECURITY SYSTEMS

"Physician's office destroyed by fire," "Dental office burglarized, set afire," "Doctor and staff held up at gunpoint"—disturbing headlines like these are all-too-frequent, but there are steps you can take to avoid having one written about you. As you plan your office, keep in mind your security needs. I've separated the dangers into three broad areas: fire, crime during office hours, and crime after office hours.

FIRE

Most fire hazards can be prevented or minimized by proper planning.

Fire from smoldering cigarettes can be prevented by prohibiting smoking in the office and by having an urn near the entry with an appropriate sign posted above it.

You can prevent some electrical fires by providing enough outlets to minimize use of extension cords.

Chances of an electrical fire starting in your office after hours will be reduced if you install and use a master electrical shut-off, as discussed in Chapter 24.

Surfaces on which Bunsen burners or ovens are to be used should be made of noncombustible material.

If you intend to keep oxygen and other gases in the office, be aware of their fire dangers. For example, *never* store or use grease or oil near the valve of an oxygen tank.

Fire can occur when the office is occupied. You should have several large fire extinguishers. Suitable locations for them include the lab, the staff lounge (particularly if any cooking is done there), and near the business office. Get the newer models that are rated A, B, and C. This means they can be used for any type of fire (wood/paper, oil, or electrical).

Telephones in the office should have, prominently displayed, the phone number of the local fire department—along with that of the police and ambulance service.

Plan for at least one alternative escape route from the office in case of fire.

Fire detection and the preservation of important records are greater problems when the office is empty than when it's occupied. To meet these problems, you need a means of notifying the fire department—and other people in the building, if any—that a fire has started and you must find a way to protect those records that would be most difficult to replace. A discussion of fire-alarm systems can be found below.

As you think about protecting important records from fire, ask yourself what records would be most difficult and/or costly to replace. On your list will probably be the following:

☐ accounts receivable and patient ledger cards;

☐ the appointment book;

☐ checkbooks and recently canceled checks;

☐ other business records and tax returns; and

☐ patient records, radiographs, and other information relating to diagnosis and treatment.

The next question is: How much money are you willing to spend to safeguard these items?

The least expensive safeguard for valuable business papers is a fireproof file cabinet. We use a four-drawer legal-size file cabinet (cost in 1980: about $700), which holds all of our recent business records and our appointment book. It's rated to withstand a temperature of 1,300°F for one hour without damage to the items inside. An inviolable rule in our office requires that those items that are removed from this file daily, such as ledger cards and the appointment book, are replaced whenever everyone leaves the office, and the drawers are closed.

We use two additional safeguards for our accounts receivable and appointment book, since if a fire burns long enough and hot enough, even a fireproof file cabinet is vulnerable.

Since we use a photocopy billing system, one of our assistants periodically makes an extra copy of every ledger card. One of us takes the copies home. Although these "fire copies" are not updated as frequently as a computer service bureau's records are, they'd permit reconstructing most of what is owed to us, when combined with our *telephone lists*, our final safeguard.

The part of the northeast where we practice is subject to winter storms and icy roads. Years ago, I developed a system of taking home each night during the winter months a copy of the following day's patient list. The ones we post around the office show patients' names and the procedures that are to be performed that day. But the one I took home also had each patient's phone number listed on it. If the driving conditions were bad enough next day to prevent my getting in to the office on time, I was able to call the patients to arrange new appointments.

I soon realized that this system, used now year-round, gave us a complete and up-to-date list of all our patients. My partner or I save these sheets at home for a year or more. If a catastrophe were to demolish our office, a reconstruction of our patient lists would still be possible from the accumulated day sheets.

(For a small additional premium, you can add *records insurance* to your office fire policy. This provides funds for the extra clerical help you'd need to reassemble records.)

Safeguarding patient records from fire is a separate and more difficult problem. The use of many fireproof file cabinets is impractical for holding thousands of folders. In addition to their cost, these cabinets are so heavy (a single four-drawer file may weigh up to 600 pounds empty) that most office floors would require massive and very expensive reinforcement to support a large number of them.

A second possibility is the use of microfilm or photocopying to make copies of records for storage outside the office. Besides cost, the disadvantages of microfilming include the need for updating the copies regularly and the difficulty of copying radiographs.

CRIME PREVENTION DURING WORKING HOURS

The thought of an intruder entering your office to rob and possibly assault is frightening. It's more of a problem when a single staff member, such as your secretary, must work alone at times in the office. Depending on your office location, the number of tenants in the building, and other factors, you may or may not have to think of security systems.

Here are a few ideas to make your office more secure:

1. Install an electric latch on the door to your office, with the button that operates the release located at your secretary's desk. An intercom from the secretary's desk to the hall outside the door can permit her to learn the identity of a visitor. The office door can have what is known as a schoolroom lock. When unlocked, the knob can be turned and the door opened from either side. When the door is locked with a key, it can still be opened from inside by just turning the knob. (This permits an easy exit in case of fire.) But someone outside trying to get in must either have a key or must wait for the secretary to activate the electric latch release.

We have a vestibule between the building's front entry and our office entrance. Anyone who enters this vestibule from the street can be seen from the secretary's desk through a small fixed window (see Figure 41-3).

2. Arrange to have a door that can be locked between the waiting room and the rest of the office. We often close and lock such a door at lunchtime. Early arrivals for afternoon appointments can enter the waiting room through the open outer door, yet staff members who are having lunch or relaxing in other parts of the office are not disturbed. Also, when the secretary is alone in the office, the same arrangement permits the entry of the letter carrier or delivery people to the waiting room only.

3. The benefits of a panic alarm (one that sounds at the touch of a button) are debatable. It may frighten away an intruder, but it may also anger him enough to turn a nonviolent confrontation into a violent one. For that reason, a silent panic alarm may be better, one that sounds at a guard service or police headquarters.

For theft prevention during office hours:

1. Provide a secure place for staff members to keep handbags and wallets out of sight.

2. Provide a shelf and a hook (see Figure 57-4A, 4B) in each treatment room where a woman's handbag or a man's jacket can be out of the way, but always where the patient can see it. This minimizes the chance of an accusation that items from a purse or pocket disappeared while in your office.

3. Place the patients' coat rack in the waiting room where your secretary can see it.

There are other types of crime that occur during office hours, most notably embezzlement, but their prevention is related to the management of your practice rather than to office design.

CRIME WHEN THE OFFICE IS CLOSED

To stop a burglar from breaking into your office, what should you do? According to most experts, a determined professional burglar can get in and out of your office undetected, despite locks, alarms, dogs, and other deterrents.

Fortunately, the same experts say that most break-ins are the work of amateurs, not professional thieves. If you make it difficult, threatening, and time-consuming for them to enter your office, they're likely to look for easier pickings elsewhere.

Consider the following general measures while your office is in the planning stage. If you want some other specific suggestions, talk to the crime-prevention officer in your local police department.

Strong locks. Pick resistant cylinders and deadbolts aren't expensive. Good window locks force the thief to break a window to get in. He doesn't want to make that kind of noise.

Strong door frames and solid-core doors. Why use a top-grade lock if the door itself can be easily kicked in or cut through, or if the door can be pried away from a flimsy frame with a crowbar?

Window guards. Steel-mesh grates bolted to frames of basement windows can prevent entry. But don't install these where they can prevent quick escape in a fire.

Identification stickers. These are small notices you can attach to doors and windows. They state that "all items of value on these premises have been marked for identification and registered with the police"—or words to that effect. Many local police departments will supply these stickers and will lend you an engraving tool—which you can also buy for about $10—to mark an identifying number on typewriters, desk-top copiers, calculators, and other portable items. Police officials say that use of these notices improves your chances of avoiding a break-in.

Good outside lighting. If you are putting up or renovating your own building, be sure to provide adequate outside lighting on *all* sides of the building, not just in front or in the parking area (see Figure 62-2). A timer or photoelectric switch will turn the lights on or off automatically.

ALARM SYSTEMS

The questions to ask yourself when considering burglar alarms are:

1. Do I want sensors (detection devices) at doors and windows? This is called perimeter wiring. Should I get devices to detect the presence of an intruder only after he gets inside?

2. Do I want a loud bell or siren inside and outside the building to scare off the thief? Or should I have a silent alarm that notifies the police or a private guard agency that a break-in has occurred?

3. If I use an outside alarm device, is there a neighbor close enough and reliable enough to call the police if the alarm sounds?

About fire alarms:

1. Will there be people in other parts of the building when my office is closed—such as tenants in a renovated older house—who must be alerted to the presence of fire or smoke?

2. Are there neighbors close enough to hear an outside fire-alarm bell or horn and call the fire department?

3. Can I connect my fire-alarm system directly to the fire department?

4. Do I need smoke detectors? Heat detectors? Rate-of-rise (of air temperature) detectors? Others?

For the answers to these and other questions, speak to the local police and fire chiefs. There are many different requirements in different areas. Some police departments, for example, permit hooking your burglar alarm directly to a signal board that is located in their headquarters; others do not allow this. Most alarm companies are set up to receive your alarm at their central stations and then notify the police. Depending on the size of your building and the number of occupants, you may have to install fire-alarm pull boxes in several locations in addition to smoke and heat detectors. Get this information before you talk to alarm companies.

Your best bet for purchase, installation, and later servicing of your alarms is a local alarm company. As with any merchandise for which service will be needed later, the company's track record is important. Ask for suggested systems and bids from several companies. For each, get a list of local customers and call to ask about their satisfaction. In many parts of the country, alarm installers aren't licensed or otherwise regulated, so be careful about who does the job.

Ask your insurance agent about the discount offered on your fire and burglary insurance if you install alarm systems. To get the discount, you may need a system that uses UL-listed equipment and wiring techniques. This makes the system more expensive, but it's probably worth it.

Alarm companies have two basic approaches for providing their systems. They may offer you a lease-purchase arrangement under which you pay a flat amount per month for three or more years. This includes parts and labor, if service is needed, plus periodic testing. Under this system, they own the equipment throughout the full term of the lease. The chief advantage is that you don't have to pay a large amount of cash at a time when you have many other expenses.

If pressed, however, most companies also offer an outright purchase arrangement that may include parts, labor, and inspection for six months or a year. You can then get a service contract after the warranty expires. I suggest that you get full cost figures from several companies before you decide. (You can find a discussion of leasing in Chapter 11.)

Be prepared to spend several thousand dollars for even simple fire- and burglary-alarm systems, especially if much wiring is needed where access is difficult, or if sophisticated burglar-alarm equipment is used.

Can you do it yourself and save money? The answer is a qualified Yes.

Alarm equipment and wire are available in stores in most large cities (check the Yellow Pages) and also by mail order. If the systems you propose using are not too complex, you may be able to install them yourself. Be sure that you know the proper techniques. They're not too difficult if the walls are open during construction. There are many books that can show you how.

But you'll have to be there at the proper time in the construction sequence, and you'll have to finish promptly to avoid delaying the builder. Also, if you do the job, you'll have to test the system periodically and service it yourself. If it doesn't work properly, you'll have to be prepared to spend time doing a differential diagnosis.

Replacement parts are not always easy to find. At least one major manufacturer sells parts only to professional alarm installers who order on their business letterhead.

Our fire and burglar alarms were installed by two electricians who were experienced in alarm installation. They worked on weekends when they and the other workmen wouldn't interfere with each other. We regularly test the finished systems ourselves, but they are available for servicing when needed. They also did the wiring for some of our other low-voltage electrical devices: among them the assistant call system, the background music system, and the water alarm.

32

BACKGROUND MUSIC SYSTEMS

If you're planning to have "acoustic perfume" in the office, here are a few questions to think about:

1. What music source will you use? The simplest and least expensive is FM radio, but you can use cassette tapes, eight-track tapes, records, AM radio or a piped-in system. If tapes or records appeal to you, you should be aware that those you buy in local stores are meant for home use only. If you use them in an office, you could run afoul of the copyright law. While the chance of your being prosecuted may seem remote, it's still possible.

There are services that provide a fresh assortment of tapes and records each month. The materials they supply have been cleared for business use through a licensing arrangement.

2. Where will you put the tuner or player and amplifier? A good location is a closet or cabinet at or near your front office. You'll need an electric outlet inside the closet or cabinet for your power supply. You should also have some means of providing at least minimal air circulation in the enclosure to prevent heat buildup. Heat shortens the life of electronic components, although there's much less heat buildup in solid-state equipment than with the old tube types. In a wall-hung cabinet, for example, have openings drilled in top and bottom. You may, of course, simply place the equipment out in the open on a shelf. The important thing is to decide on the location now, so that the wires to your speakers can be placed in the wall nearby.

3. How many rooms will have speakers? This question is important because it relates to the type of equipment you should buy. If you'll have no more than four or five rooms with speakers, you can use ordinary hi-fi equipment with a volume control (called an L-pad) controlling the speaker in each room. However, if your office is large, with many speakers, you may find a falling off of

volume at the more distant speakers and a change in volume at some speakers as others are turned up or down.

The solution is to use a public-address amplifier. Such a device receives the signal from your tuner or tape player, amplifies it, and then sends it out to the speakers superimposed on a 25-volt or 70-volt constant voltage (C.V.). This means that all speakers receive identical power and the volume can be altered on one without affecting the others.

To use this system, each room needs a *matching transformer*—either 25- or 70-volt, depending on which C.V. is used. This converts the signal back to a form suited to the speaker. Such transformers cost about $10 to $15 each. The P.A. amplifier may cost $125 or more. These figures are in addition to the costs of tuner or tape player, volume controls, speakers, and labor. Inexpensive equipment is available at electronic parts stores. You don't need a powerful amplifier, either. Our 10-speaker system uses a 35-watt amplifier. It produces more than enough power, since we keep the music volume low. For that reason, also, we can use inexpensive speakers.

One added benefit of the amplifier: In a large office, you can connect a microphone to it and use it for paging.

Figure 32-1 is a block diagram of the wiring arrangement for a system using a P.A. amplifier.

4. Where will your speakers be located?

The usual place is above the acoustic ceiling with a grille plate covering the opening cut in the acoustic panel. We found a more unobtrusive way. We drilled a pattern of holes in a piece of pegboard. We used the pegboard as a template for drilling the ceiling panels that were to support the speakers. Each speaker was then screwed to the top surface of its panel above the holes.

The effect is one of music coming from nowhere. The irregular surface of the acoustic ceiling effectively camouflages the drilled holes (Figure 32-2).

5. Where will you install your volume controls? Choose a wall location and height in each room easily accessible to you from the spot in which you'll normally be working (see Figure 42-1).

Be sure that whoever is to install the system is provided with a floor plan that shows exactly where each component is to be placed.

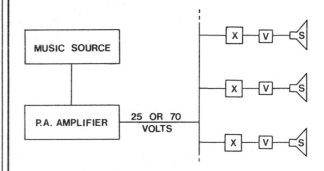

Figure 32-1. Block diagram of background music system using public-address amplifier (each line in diagram is actually a pair of wires). Music source most often is FM radio, but could be tape or record player. Most P.A. amplifiers have two C.V. (constant voltage) outputs: 25 and 70 volts. Use either one. Buy line-matching transformers (X) designed for that voltage, one for each speaker. If individual volume controls (V), are used, install one in each room between transformer and speaker. See text for advantages of such a system over usual hi-fi setup.

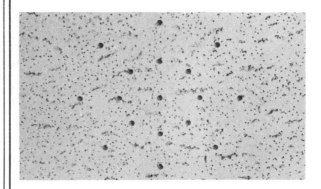

Figure 32-2. Holes in acoustic ceiling panel eliminate need for special grille plate. Speaker is mounted on upper side of panel. Pattern and size (one-quarter inch) of holes were decided arbitrarily. A template, made from pegboard, guided drilling of the holes.

33
HARDWARE

Locks, keys, hinges, and sliding tracks are items that we ordinarily don't think much about. But they're extremely important to plan for in terms of both security and convenience.

In Chapter 31, I described the electric latch and the schoolroom lock for the office-entry door. Other doors that need locks are lavatories and the darkroom. You may want also to lock storage closets and your private office.

If your rented office is in a commercial or professional office building and the construction is being done by the landlord, you'll be offered the *building standard* hardware. The term (used for other building materials also) means a quality of hardware that is standard for that building. If you want a better, more attractive grade you'll pay extra for it.

Your best bet is probably the building standard hardware for most knobs, locks, and hinges if they look reasonably attractive. The items that should be the finest obtainable are sliding-door hardware, especially if you're using heavy solid-core doors, and the locks for the outer doors of the office. Other items that should be planned for are door closers, kickplates, door bumpers, and a mail slot.

If you are an owner of a new building being designed, you should discuss hardware with the architect before the final plans and specifications are prepared. Give some thought to keying arrangements: Which doors should be keyed alike; which should have access only by a separate key; how many master keys do you need and for whom should they be made?

VI
THE FINAL STAGES OF PLANNING

34
FINAL PLANS AND SPECIFICATIONS

The *working drawings* are the culmination of your weeks or months of plans, discussions, revisions, and more discussions and revisions. They should be identical to the last revision of your preliminary plans, but with enough added detail, so that from them a builder will be able to offer a comprehensive bid for the entire job.

THE OFFICE'S FINAL PLANS

When you get the final office plans from the architect, take plenty of time to review them carefully. Be sure that you understand all the abbreviations. If you're not sure, *ask*—even if you've asked the same question several times before. Why? Because this is your last chance to make changes without extra cost. A shift in the location of a door or in the placement of a sink, for example, can usually be managed even if other changes must also be made as a result. Try to do this after the contract has been signed and you'll find yourself with big bills for extras.

There's another reason to go over every page carefully. Architects, like doctors, are human. Mistakes, omissions, and misunderstandings occur. Catch them early and avoid the grief later.

WHAT TO LOOK FOR

If your new office doesn't require extensive construction, some of the drawings discussed here won't concern you. But you must be prepared to deal with a few of these in any case.

The floor plan shows location of partitions and doors and the direction of door swings. Are they all correct?

Interior elevations show a front view of those walls that are unusual in some respect, such as one that has a passthrough. They may be needed to show changes in floor or ceiling levels.

Sections and details show the particulars of special features, such as the soundproofing of a partition, or the location of a particular mechanical item, such as a valve.

The plumbing plan is a copy of the floor plan with all sinks and toilets shown as well as the location of the compressor, central suction, and other plumbing items. The approximate location of the pipes going to equipment will also be shown, but the exact arrangement of pipes will be set by a template of the junction box to be supplied by your equipment dealer.

Where special work is needed to support a plumbing fixture, it should be noted. For example, if you select a toilet that will hang on the wall (rather than standing on the floor), that wall will need reinforcement. A schedule of plumbing fixtures to be supplied by the builder, including type, manufacturer, and size, should be available with the plumbing plan.

The electrical plan will specify details of the electrical service, its metering, and safety features. Location and height of all duplex wall outlets should be shown, as well as the location of all fixtures and the switches that control them. Location and details of special circuits, such as for X-ray equipment, examining table, or dental chair, should be noted. A schedule of lighting fixtures accompanying the electrical plan should show catalog number and manufacturer plus the type and quantity of lamps used. Suggestion: Specify that each fixture is to be supplied with lamps. The builder will probably get them at a better price than you can.

The final electrical plan should not be considered final until all decisions are made about furniture and built-ins that might influence outlet location and lighting. The placement of desks, file cabinets, and treatment-room countertops, for example, will determine where the accompanying electrical and telephone outlets should be.

A series of schedules should come with the final plans. These should list doors, windows, hardware, wall finishes, and floor finishes. For each item, the architect should list the pertinent features. The door schedule, for example, should show each door's type (solid or hollow or louver), thickness, size, and other details. If an item, such as carpeting, won't be supplied by the general contractor, it still should be noted in the schedules, because the builder must know how to prepare the underlying floor.

A separate plan may be drawn by the architect or interior designer showing the furniture and built-ins—sometimes called *casework*—superimposed on the floor plan. This may or may not be included with the working drawings, depending on whether the builder or an outside contractor is to supply the built-ins. Using a copy of the floor plan insures that the furniture will fit.

Note this point: Where a piece of furniture or office equipment, such as a file cabinet, must fit into a space with little room to spare, the size of the space needed should be written by the architect on the floor plan. In other words, don't rely just on the scale of the plans. Writing in the crucial dimension will direct the carpenter's attention to it. If he overlooks it, it's his problem to correct, not yours. As we'll discuss in Chapter 47, during construction you'll have to be alert to whether the plans are being followed.

Accompanying your working drawings should be a series of typewritten pages called *specifications*, usually spoken of as the *specs*. They set the performance standards for the work in terms of administration, time, construction, adequacy, and general working conditions. Their purpose is to explain those details that are not apparent from the drawings alone. They include the grades of materials, how they are to be installed, and the quality of workmanship expected. The specs should include any special installation requirements, provided by your supplier, for your equipment and special procedures, such as pressure testing of nitrous oxide and oxygen lines.

The working drawings and specifications are considered *contract documents*. They are part of your contract with the builder.

THE BUILDING'S FINAL PLANS

The working drawings for a building are much more complex than those for an office. Elevations show its outward appearance on all sides. Sections show how the foundation is to be built and how various areas relate to those above and below them. Details illustrate how decorative items are to be built. In a larger building, structural and mechanical engineering drawings show the steel work and the heating, ventilating, and air-conditioning particulars. Outside, separate drawings show the blacktopped parking area with its *birms* (curbs) and walks. A landscape plan may show what trees and shrubs are to be planted and where grass or ground covers are called for.

Should you be concerned with every detail on every page? No, not unless you're really interested enough to spend the time learning the terminology. I suggested above that you should scrutinize every item on your office plans. You'll be intimately and constantly involved with how every part of the office functions. In a large building, however, the structural and mechanical details can be overwhelming. If you've chosen your architect wisely, rely on him.

This doesn't mean you should give the final plans just a casual glance, either. In a small building, particularly, the plans and specs of the building include those of your own office, so you'll have to look at them carefully. If you're erecting a multioffice structure, however, each office is likely to be shown just as an open suite, with separate plans for its construction.

The portions of the building's final drawings that should interest you most are the outside elevations, the drawings of the lobby and hallways, the site plan, and the landscaping plans. These are what will be seen and used by visitors to your building. They will have a major influence on how desirable your building will be to prospective tenants and, at some time in the future, to a purchaser. This will be your last chance to make meaningful changes without excessive cost.

WHAT TO LOOK FOR

Elevations. Has the architect caught the spirit you agreed on in your early discussions? Have the changes agreed upon at later meetings been made? Are you satisfied with the front entry's appearance? Do the windows and the roof line harmonize with the rest of the building? Have you seen samples of the exterior materials to be used?

Have you looked closely at the *rear* elevation of the building? If patients will have to drive around the building when entering or leaving, you'll want the back to look presentable. Where will trash bins be kept? Will a garbage truck emptying these bins block traffic around the building?

Floor plan. Is the lobby spacious enough? Will it be well lit with natural or artificial light? Will it have some attractive decorative features, such as plants or sculptures, to keep it from being stark? Will the hallways be comfortably wide and well lit?

Site plan. The parking and driveway arrangement will be your chief concern. Will the cars enter and leave your property easily? Does the pattern of parking —curbside, diagonal, or perpendicular—make sense?

Specifications. The specs for even a medium-sized building can easily be thicker than your local phone book. If you read through them, your reaction may be that they tell you more than you want to know.

Ask the architect if the specs require the builder to submit "as-built" drawings before receiving his final payment. This is a set of drawings that show the locations of all pipes and ducts and the direction of flow in each. They can be important later if repairs or additions are needed.

Landscaping plan. It's desirable to have a landscaping plan completed by this stage, but it doesn't always happen. Landscaping plans aren't really part of the final plans and specs because a separate contractor is usually involved.

Have you selected the landscape architect (if one is needed) and the plant nursery with as much care as you put into the choice of other experts? Landscaping is an integral part of office building construction. The clean lines and good looks of a building lose much of their appeal if the building is surrounded by poorly chosen plantings.

Has the landscaping been planned to require minimum maintenance? Labor is expensive. If a fairly large expanse is to be covered with greenery, consider ground covers rather than lawns.

Do you understand clearly what the nurseryman will and will not do? Ask him to list specifically, before signing a contract, what soil preparation procedures he'll perform and what will be your (or your general contractor's) responsibility. For example, unless it's part of the contract, the nursery won't do any machine grading or removal of debris or large rocks. If you're not clear about these details you could be presented with a bill for extra work later.

Are you acquainted with the kinds of plants and trees being recommended? Better see them in the sizes recommended before agreeing to their use. Have you checked with the building inspector to find out if the community limits the height of shrubs or other plantings. Some do.

Shrub sizes are usually specified by their height above the ground. Trees are measured by their *caliper,* the diameter of the trunk at a point four feet above the ground.

35

BUILDERS, BIDS, AND CONTRACTS

Your plans and specs are finished. On paper, everything looks great. Now you have to get it built in a reasonable time and at a reasonable cost.

In many earlier chapters, I've treated the office and building separately, since the concerns were often different. Here, I discuss them together, because the issues—selecting builders, obtaining bids, agreeing to a contract—are the same. They differ mainly in the dollar amounts involved.

One question often arises: Should you be your own general contractor (G.C.)? My answer is *No*, not unless you've worked in the building trades before and the project is a small one. For a large office or an entire building, you'll take so much time away from your practice that any anticipated savings will evaporate.

There are other problems, too. If you are your own G.C., you will have to find 100 percent financing, which is unlikely, or else advance your own cash to get the project started. You'll find difficulty in buying materials at the prices regular contractors can obtain. You'll have no recourse to anyone else if things go wrong. Finally, you'll need extra liability insurance against mishaps on the job. Since you're not a recognized builder, this may be difficult to find.

FINDING A GENERAL CONTRACTOR

The two best sources for finding builders to bid on your project are your architect and other doctors. A third may be your equipment dealer. Wherever the recommendation comes from, do some further checking on your own. This first inquiry need not be an intensive investigation. Right now you're interested only in whether it's worthwhile asking a particular builder to bid on your job.

Your architect will prepare several sets of plans and specs (which you'll pay for) to be picked up by the builders you've selected. Try to find three or four possible contractors. Their bids should give you a realistic idea of what the project's cost will be. If you ask for a price from only one, you won't know whether he's high or low.

The specs should specify a deadline for the bid, what levels of insurance coverage the builder is expected to have, and other general requirements.

Depending on the size of the job, the bidders could need from a few days to six weeks to review all the documents and submit bids. During that time, all you can do is wait and hope for the best.

As the bids come in, you'll find out how good your architect was at estimating costs. Typically, most reputable builders submit bids that are fairly close (within 10 percent or so) to one another. If one bid is substantially higher than the rest, it could be because the builder isn't interested in getting the contract or he doesn't understand what is involved. He'll do the job only if the profit margin is sweetened.

An exceptionally low bid must be looked at carefully. It may mean that this builder is desperate for this job or that he's overlooked something important in the plans or specs. In either case, he's likely to cut corners in labor or materials to come out of the project with a profit. If he's overlooked an important item, he may come to you or to your architect when the job is half finished with a tale of woe about his error.

What will you do then? One choice will be to insist on his honoring the contract to the letter. But to do this can force him into an insolvent position. He may walk off the job to cut his losses. Threats to sue will be fruitless, since he'll have few assets to lose and a lawsuit will take several years.

Another alternative—and a more likely one—will be to pay him an additional amount to compensate for the work he overlooked. This may bring his bid close to, or even higher than, those of other bidders.

There are some good builders who can submit low bids because they work with lower overhead than others. If you're lucky enough to find such a gem, as we were, grab him! They are likely to be small firms in which the principals are themselves in one of the building trades. In our case, the builders were both carpenters.

Your safest bet may be to eliminate both very high and very low bidders and accept one in the middle. Unfortunately, a frequent problem is that all of the bids are far higher than anticipated. Your choices, if this happens, are to:

☐ rage at your architect, dismiss him, and find another—a satisfying approach, but likely to cause delays;

☐ invite bids from another group of builders, though these aren't likely to be too different from the first;

☐ pick out one builder who seems reasonable, and let the architect meet with him to find those areas where costs can be reduced;

☐ ask the architect to revise the plans to make the work less expensive; or

☐ swallow hard and agree to the higher cost.

This is one of those moments that justify all the time spent months earlier to find the right architect. If you have a good one, he'll have previously identified those aspects of the project that are likely to increase the cost substantially, and where cuts can be made.

The most likely outcome of this particular trauma will be some combination of the last three choices. Note that this sort of problem is much more likely when an entire building is under consideration rather than just interior construction for an office. The latter can be estimated with far greater accuracy.

Before you decide definitely on a builder, there is more investigation to be done. Speak first to those doctors for whom he's worked:

☐ Were they satisfied with his workmanship?

☐ Did he complete the job without excessive delays?

☐ Were his bills for extra work fair?

☐ Did he return promptly during the warranty period to correct any problems?

☐ Would they engage him again for another job?

While these inquiries are going on, have the builder's credit checked. You or your lawyer can get a report from the local credit bureau on his company. You should be interested in:

☐ how long this particular company has been in existence (a recently formed company could mean that his previous corporation went bankrupt);

☐ whether any lawsuits are pending against the company and by whom; and
☐ whether there are any outstanding judgments or liens.

I suggest that such a credit check be made even if the job is relatively small. An insolvent builder can cause considerable delay and expense if he goes bankrupt in the middle of your job and you suddenly have to find a new G.C.

One final call should be made to the Better Business Bureau. You'll want to know if they've had complaints about this builder or his company.

The process just described is known as *lump-sum* or *fixed-price* contracting. It's probably the best kind of arrangement for you, since you know in advance what you'll be called on to pay. Another type of agreement is known as a *time-and-materials* or *cost-plus* contract. It works this way: You select a reputable contractor who proposes an upset (maximum) price for the job. He then does the work and charges labor and materials costs plus an agreed-upon additional percentage for his overhead and profit. If the final figure is below the upset price, you benefit from the savings (or you and the contractor share the savings). If the costs go over the upset price, he pays the excess amount.

Avoid such a contract if you can. It usually costs more than a fixed-price arrangement. Sometimes, however, the uncertainties inherent in a job, such as the renovation of an old building, make such a contract the only kind a builder will accept.

The remainder of this chapter discusses the details of only the lump-sum type of contract, which was the kind we used.

COMPLETION DATE

You want your office as soon as possible. You've heard friends tell horror stories about months of delays when they built their offices. You're determined not to let this happen to you. What should you do?

Let the builder and the architect work out an anticipated completion date, but don't take that date seriously. It may surprise you to learn that the builder will be just as anxious as you are about finishing the work. He won't get his profit out of the project until your last payment is made.

The building trades are notorious for delays. The builder is at the mercy of strikes, late deliveries, and assorted work stoppages. Delays on your job cost him money. He'll have borrowed money to buy materials and pay his work-men; he'll repay his note only as you pay him.

There are some unscrupulous builders who start more jobs than they can handle in order not to miss any contracts. If you're involved with one of these you're in trouble. That's why I urge you to investigate carefully the builder's past record, reputation, and solvency.

PAYMENTS

Don't pay *anything* in advance. Payments in most commercial construction are made as the work progresses. You should discuss this with your architect before negotiating with the builder.

The usual method is a monthly payment based on the amount of work completed. If the job is small, the payments may be made at shorter intervals.

On our project it worked this way: At the end of each month the builder submitted a standard A.I.A. requisition for payment to the architect, who visited the site. If the work completed was as claimed, the architect approved the requisition and sent copies to us and to our bank's appraiser. The appraiser visited the site to verify the work independently. He notified the bank that we were entitled to a portion of our construction loan. We then used this money to pay the builder.

Each payment was for the amount approved by the architect *less 10 percent*. This amount held back from each payment is called *retainage*. Its purpose is to assure that the work is completed properly. The accumulated retainage is not paid until several weeks—the exact time is stipulated in the contract—after the job has reached what is known as *substantial completion* as verified by the architect.

(This retainage is not the same as a *construction holdback*. The latter, mentioned in Chapter 18, is a lender's insistence on withholding part of your loan until you have leases for a specified percentage of the building's rentable space.)

This method of payment is for the owner's protection, and you should insist on it. The reason is that if, for any reason, the builder cannot or will not complete the work, you can use the retainage to get it done by someone else.

PENALTY CLAUSES

The idea of exacting a penalty from the builder for every day the job is delayed past the agreed-upon completion time seems attractive at first glance. But don't even try it. Penalty clauses are rarely enforceable.

If you insist on one, the builder will defer his completion date to one he knows he can fulfill, or he'll find loopholes in the contract to avoid the penalty, or he'll insist on a bonus for each day he finishes ahead of schedule.

The old proverb "You'll catch more flies with honey than with vinegar" applies here. If you must get your office finished by a certain date, offer the bonus alone. If it's at all possible for the contractor to meet that deadline, the added incentive will probably do the trick; if the delay is beyond his control, no penalty, however severe, will work. Furthermore, if you have a penalty clause and the work exceeds the completion date by many days, the total dollar amount of the penalty can be higher than the builder's profit. He may then just abandon the job unless you agree to drop the penalty.

UNIT COSTS AND EXTRAS

If your project is a large and complicated one, especially if you're creating a building, you should try to come to an understanding with the builder *before* the contract is signed about items that may not yet be shown on the drawings. For example, if your plans and specs for the building shell are complete, but some of the individual offices have not yet been fully designed, your architect should obtain *unit costs* from the builder. These might include dollar amounts:

☐ per electric outlet (in the construction industry the word outlet means any location where wires come out of a wall; this could be a duplex receptacle, a light fixture, or a wall switch);

☐ per fluorescent fixture;

☐ per separate circuit;

☐ per sink including supply lines and waste; and

☐ per linear foot of partition.

In this way, you'll know in advance what these elements will cost even if the total dollar amount is still uncertain.

When the builder provides these figures, you may be in a position to negotiate some of the prices. At this stage, the builder will try to keep the amounts low because he still doesn't have a signed contract in his pocket. In effect, he'll often agree to charge you his wholesale price for some of these items because he expects to make enough of a profit on the large job.

Once the contract is signed and work is under way, however, the picture changes. If you now ask for something extra to be done, the price is likely to be "T and M plus 15 and 10." This means time (the charge for labor) plus materials (at full price) plus 15 percent (for the builder's overhead) plus 10 percent or more (for profit). When figured in this way, the unit cost for the item will be much higher than it might have been if negotiated earlier. Some unscrupulous builders have been known to inflate prices exorbitantly for previously overlooked extras, knowing that unless the particular item, such as special soundproofing, for example, is installed at that point during construction its cost will be prohibitive later on. You can avoid such unpleasantness by selecting your builder with care, by thinking out the details of your own office thoroughly in advance with the full participation and control of the architect, and by obtaining unit costs where appropriate before signing the contract.

ALLOWANCES

There are certain items, usually *finish* materials, such as carpeting, floor tiles, light fixtures, and hardware, that come in a wide range of grades and styles from many sources. You may want to order these yourself or through your architect or interior designer rather than through the builder.

A frequent practice is to provide an allowance in the contract for such articles. The allowance will usually pay for a low grade of the item and the builder will provide it if you wish. If you obtain a better grade yourself, you'll pay for it directly and deduct the allowance from the amount owed to the builder.

This approach is to your advantage, since it makes the contractor responsible for the installation of the item no matter who provides it.

36
THE TIMING OF CONSTRUCTION

I mentioned in the previous chapter that estimates of how long construction is likely to take can be notoriously inaccurate. Yet some estimates will obviously be necessary, since equipment and furniture dealers must be given a target date for deliveries.

My own experience and that of other doctors has been that for a small building, a reasonable estimate of the time needed is six months (plus or minus two) from ground breaking to move-in.

For interior construction alone, as in a leased office, the time involved can range from four weeks to four months or more, despite frequent builder promises of needing "just a few weeks."

Does it have to be that way? Not necessarily, but in my part of the country, at least, I have never heard of an office construction job that was finished when promised. The main reasons for delay are these:

1. Deliveries are often late. If the delayed item is one that must be installed before others can be put in, its absence can cause the whole job to stop. For example, the lead for lining walls is often supplied attached to panels of wallboard. These are installed in the same manner as regular wallboard. If the leaded wallboard is delayed, it means that the spacklers—the workers who tape and fill the seams and nail holes—cannot complete their job. This, in turn, means that the painting or papering can't be done.

2. Another source of delay is the sequencing of the various trades. If the electrician and plumber have not finished their *rough-ins*—the installation of the principal wires and pipes that go inside the walls and above the ceiling—the wallboard and ceiling installers cannot do their work. Most building tradesmen juggle several jobs at once. If your plumber is held up on another job, his absence can delay all of the trades whose work comes after his.

There is no way to beat this problem. All you can do is be aware that such delays are common and to expect them. It'll help if you have selected all equipment needing special wiring or plumbing before construction starts. Your equipment supplier will provide templates showing what pipes and wires are needed and where; one significant source of delay will have been avoided.

Most of the workmen who'll be building your office in the early stages will be employees of the contractor or subcontractors. These tradesmen will be called in as needed by the builders. Later, however, you'll have to arrange for some installations and deliveries yourself, so you'll have to keep abreast of what's happening each week and what's to happen in the near future. Here are some examples:

1. After the framing is finished, but before the walls are closed up with wall-board, your telephone installer should put in his cables. You'll have to tell him when he can come in. Similarly, you'll have to plan the wiring for your burglar- and/or fire-alarm systems, music system, and signaling systems if these are to be done by outside contractors or by yourself.

2. Near the end of the job, when most of the construction and mechanical work is done, you'll have to work out the sequence for the finishing steps. A reasonable sequence will be: priming and painting of walls, followed by paperhanging and installation of vinyl wall covering; next, floor coverings (carpet or vinyl) can go in; then your equipment and furniture can be delivered and installed.

Although each stage needs only a few days, the workers may not be available when you need them, so at least a week can be spent for each step.

The best advice is to start early enough and be patient. Above all, get each step done right the first time through.

VII
DECORATING, FURNITURE, AND EQUIPMENT

37
THE OFFICE ATMOSPHERE

The philosophy that guided us in furnishing and decorating our office is this: Many patients coming to a doctor's office—any kind of doctor—are anxious about pain, about what dire things the doctor may tell them, or about cost. The office, we feel, should be planned to be as nonthreatening as possible to keep this anxiety level to a minimum. Some of the techniques we use are subliminal. Patients feel more comfortable without realizing why. We want to transmit this message, even though we don't say it in so many words: "Welcome to our office. We're pleased that you've chosen us to care for you. We'll do our best to help you."

Our effort to produce this kind of atmosphere takes many forms. I've listed them here as a series of suggestions for you to consider.

1. Your office should *not* be decorated and furnished as if it were your home. Your home's decor should please you and your family, but your office must have a more universal appeal. You need not just good taste, but good taste combined with an understanding of its effect on others.

2. Emphasize soft and rounded shapes in your furnishings rather than hard, sharp ones. Angular forms suggest painful stimuli and create uneasiness.

3. Select colors for your floors, walls, and furniture that are restful and pleasing to most people. The earth tones we used—mostly beiges, browns, oranges, and wood grains—draw continuing compliments from patients and visitors to the office.

4. Choose colors in your art objects that blend with the color scheme in the rest of the office.

5. Your office should have an uncluttered look. This is one more reason to be sure that you get enough space. When people, furniture, and equipment are jammed together, the effect is disquieting.

6. Keep the air in the office fresh and free of strange or unpleasant odors. Proper ventilation and a "No Smoking" rule will help.

7. Use appropriate lighting levels for each part of the office. In particular, avoid placing light sources where they shine directly into patients' eyes.

8. Control the sound level by using background music, acoustic ceilings, remote placement of noise-producing equipment, and the other techniques discussed in Chapter 27.

9. Select textures in your furniture that are pleasing to touch.

10. Maintain comfortable temperatures in all rooms.

11. When patients must remain in one position for a long time, as in a treatment room, give them something interesting to look at rather than a blank wall or ceiling. Possibilities include macramé plant hangers, decorative pots and plants, mobiles, sculpture, needlepoint hangings, graphics, and paintings (see Figure 57-1A).

12. Be certain that the patients' lavatory is always kept neat, clean, and well-supplied with toilet tissue, paper towels, and paper cups. The wastebasket should be emptied frequently. Don't make the room too elaborate, though. You won't want patients spending excessive amounts of time there.

13. Employ staff members with ready smiles, pleasant voices, and friendly personalities. Insist that they wear clean, well-fitting uniforms in colors that don't clash with other colors in the office. While this is not strictly a function of office design, it contributes so strongly to the office's atmosphere that it's worth mentioning. A sloppy, grouchy, carelessly dressed, or inconsiderate assistant can undo all of your other efforts to reassure an anxious patient.

All of these conscious efforts to create a comfortable atmosphere for patients will have similar effects on your staff and yourself. When you practice in your well-planned new office, you should expect to work more efficiently, under reduced stress, and to come home at night feeling more relaxed and less tired. You should find, as we do, that this adds enormously to your satisfaction with your new surroundings.

(See Chapter 57 for additional suggestions for creating a pleasant office atmosphere.)

38
INTERIOR DESIGN
AND DESIGNERS

The details of your office that your patients will notice more than any other are its interior design features. Your furniture, carpeting, wall coverings, accessories, and art work all create the office's atmosphere.

A pleasing, reassuring atmosphere doesn't spring up by hit-or-miss purchases. It needs as much conscious planning as any other part of your office. And as with the rest of your office, you'll make fewer mistakes if you have a professional guiding you.

But be careful: There are several different categories of people who call themselves *interior designers*.

At the top is the person who belongs to the American Society of Interior Designers, who uses the initials A.S.I.D. after his name, and who works independently, not directly affiliated with any store or manufacturer. Membership in the A.S.I.D. requires some rigorous testing, including portfolios of past work. The group is trying hard to upgrade the standards in this field. The designer will sell you his services by the hour (range: $30 to $100 per hour) or for a lump sum negotiated in advance, sometimes based on the size of the office ($1 to $1.50 or more per square foot).

You may also order your furniture through the designer, who can usually get a better discount than you can. The designer acts as a middleman in the transaction. For example, if the furniture article's list price is $1,000 and the designer's discount is 40 percent, he pays $600. You may pay the designer $700 or $800 for the article (although some of the very top designers will charge you the full price of $1,000).

The interior designer may also serve as your space planner. There are some in this field who specialize in professional office layout and planning. From such a designer, the services you receive include space planning and interior design rolled into one package, and his fee reflects this. Conversely, some architects double as interior designers, at least to the extent of suggesting types of furniture or carpeting and ordering it for you.

The practice of the designer's charging a fee for design services apart from any purchases is relatively recent. In the past, you were expected to buy a minimum dollar amount of furniture and accessories. The designer's services were supplied in return for his commission.

The separate fee idea has at least one major advantage. The designer will—or should—be interested only in what is best for your office, without any interest in how or where you obtain the items.

A second category of designer is the one affiliated with a furniture dealer. He sometimes doubles as a salesperson. No separate design fee is charged. This designer, who may or may not be a member of A.S.I.D., receives a commission on what you buy. He'll be interested in selling his own company's products, but can usually obtain pieces from other dealers and manufacturers as well. Such a designer sometimes works for a major supplier of professional equipment and will try to sell you a particular line of furniture.

The major problem with this group of designers is that the designer's principal interest is usually in making the sale. He may not be willing to spend much time with you to learn your needs and your likes and dislikes.

A third major category of designers, possibly the largest, I call the amateurs. These are people who enjoy choosing furniture, carpeting, and accessories and who often have a natural flair for it. Some establish a working relationship with one or more distributors, and others arrange to make their purchases through a professional designer.

Do you need an interior designer? If you think so, from which group should you choose? The best advice I can offer you is to go by the designer's past record, no matter what the person's training or affiliation.

As with many other personal services, however, you'll pretty much get what you pay for, if you spend enough time investigating. I strongly recommend engaging an independent professional designer when there are several partners involved. As I noted in Chapter 13, you'll be asking for trouble if you engage the services of a wife or relative of one of your partners as the designer.

Our experience with an interior designer left us with mixed emotions. He was affiliated with an office furniture company, but he also did independent design work. We chose him after seeing several offices he had done and receiving favorable comments about him and his work. To his credit, he focused on some of the important elements of design: scale, texture, variety, arrangement; he suggested an attractive sectional sofa for a difficult corner of our waiting room; he designed and had built a matching low bench; he took us to a furniture showroom where we selected some barrel chairs, which we like very much; he obtained the furniture as well as the carpeting and the sheet vinyl floor covering at prices that were as low as any we could expect to find.

On the negative side, he was of little help in choosing either fabrics or colors. His designs for built-in desks were unoriginal; they were mostly reworkings of our architect's suggestions. His promises of delivery were sometimes ludicrous. Some items that we expected to have in 12 weeks were delivered more than 12 months later.

The designer acted as a catalyst in many situations. Though we often did not accept his suggestions, they directed our attention to some unrecognized aspect of the problem. This led us to arrive at a satisfactory solution ourselves. For example, we chose none of the upholstery fabrics he brought for our approval, but in discussing them we found other fabrics that worked out very well. We selected vinyl wall coverings on our own, but he pointed out where certain of the textures would be better than others.

How and when do you go about selecting an interior designer? What should you expect of him?

If you plan to use the services of an architect as well as an interior designer, get the two experts together as early as possible in the planning stages. In other words, find your designer before any final decisions are made about floor plans or materials to be used.

Before you try to find a designer, you should give serious thought to the image or theme you want to project. Are you looking for a relaxed, homelike atmosphere? An antiseptic, clinical look? A dignified, traditional feeling? Space-age modernity? An image of prestige and success? If you know what you want you'll have a much better chance of getting it.

Next, look at recently decorated offices, especially those with an atmosphere similar to what you want. Find out who the designer was and talk to him. Ask to see other offices done by the same designer.

Be sure you and the designer understand each other. Is his fee structure acceptable and explicit?

Once the designer has become familiar with the floor plan of your office and with your desires—and this may require several meetings—he should be able to offer you a *design presentation*. This is the designer's concept of how the different rooms in your office should look. It should include:

☐ large-scale drawings of the rooms with the furniture drawn in;

☐ perspective drawings where needed;

☐ catalog photos of the furniture;

☐ samples of fabrics suggested for furniture and draperies, including several color choices; and

☐ samples of carpeting and wall coverings.

This meeting may be only the prelude to others as your ideas become clearer. If possible, go to showrooms with the designer to see the furniture. Try to get large pieces of proposed carpeting or wall covering. You may not be able to judge the effect of a pattern from a small swatch.

About photos and samples: I strongly advise that you *never* order any article of furniture or equipment without a clear photo or drawing that remains in your possession and shows the item's catalog number. Similarly, you should have a labeled sample of every "finish" item in its desired color—that is, every surface that will be seen in the finished office and building. This means brick, vinyl, or aluminum siding, stone, paneling, paint, stain, wallpaper, carpeting, vinyl asbestos or sheet vinyl flooring, upholstery fabric, draperies, shades, plastic laminate, ceiling tile, and any other surface.

Whenever you receive an invoice for something you've ordered, you should check the catalog numbers against your photos and samples. If you don't, you're likely to be very upset when you wait four months for delivery, only to find that the designer misunderstood your order.

Some mistakes and communication gaps are almost inevitable, but you can minimize them by taking such precautions.

39

FLOOR COVERINGS

You'll want to cover the floors in your office, and the material you'll probably think of first is carpeting. In recent years, carpeting has become the favorite because of its appearance, its softness, and its ability to muffle sounds. New techniques of dyeing man-made fibers provide almost an unlimited variety of colors and patterns to choose from.

CHOOSING CARPETING MATERIAL

What kind of carpeting material should you choose? Nylon and, to a lesser extent, polypropylene (olefin) are the most widely used synthetics in medical and dental offices. Their ease of maintenance, stain resistance, sound absorption, resistance to wear, and control of static electricity give them the edge over other types of fibers.

Many chemical companies make the synthetic fibers that are sold to the carpet manufacturers to be dyed and made into carpet. The fibers themselves are known by their trade names. For example, Antron and Anso-X are the nylon carpet fibers made by DuPont and Allied Chemical, respectively, while Herculon is the polypropylene produced by Hercules. As far as I can determine, there's little difference among the brands within a group.

Which areas should you carpet? The waiting room, hallways, front office, and private office are where carpeting is used most frequently. Many doctors are now placing it in treatment rooms and work areas, too, but this use is still controversial for several reasons.

The argument favoring carpeting in treatment rooms holds that it is soft underfoot, has a warm look, does not require costly regular waxing as does sheet vinyl or tile, and, according to the Carpet and Rug Institute, tests have shown that it is at least as sanitary as the resilient floor coverings if cleaned properly.

On the negative side, compared with vinyl flooring, carpeting reduces the ease of movement of operating stools and other furniture on casters; spills may be harder to clean up, and the surface remains damp longer; and in the dental operatory, the accumulation of mercury droplets may increase the risk of mercury toxicity.

We use sheet vinyl in our treatment rooms primarily because there are few seams and because it permits our operating stools to move somewhat more freely than they would on carpeting.

What colors, texture, and pile should you look for? Generally, tweeds or small patterns are recommended for camouflaging dirt, particularly in a waiting room where patients bring soil and grease in on their shoes from a parking lot. A *level-loop* (sometimes called *round-wire)* pile is often suggested for this kind of application. It can be used in hallways and other parts of your office as well. For your private office, however, you may want the luxurious look, feel, and sound reduction of a deep pile.

How can you select carpeting that will have a long life expectancy? Carpeting can look worn out either because the pile yarns are destroyed or because the pile yarns are intact but are matted down. You can choose a pile that does not become easily matted. The following is from the *Carpet Specifiers Handbook*, second edition, reprinted by courtesy of the Carpet and Rug Institute: "If carpeting has an adequately dense pile, grit tends to remain on the surface so that it can be vacuumed away more easily and thoroughly. At the same time, the denser the pile, the less likelihood of permanent crushing because the pile yarns will tend to support themselves in the upright position. In effect, they have no room to topple over."

A carpet that has a dense pile feels thick when you press it or step on it. Other factors related to a carpet's durability are pile height (the distance from the top of the pile to the top of the backing) and face weight (ounces per square yard). The Institute suggests: "To judge the relative quality of carpet, face weights, pile heights, and density . . . must be compared. In general, the deeper, denser, and heavier the pile—all else being equal—the better the carpet."

The carpeting we chose was an Antron III nylon. (The "III" refers to a form of Antron with built-in antistatic properties.) It's a level-loop pile with a salt-and-pepper pattern of light and dark browns. For our private office, we have a deeper-pile nylon in a solid tan-gold.

Some additional thoughts about carpeting:

1. The use of synthetic fibers, especially nylon, has kept the cost of carpeting down to acceptable levels. In 1980, the price was approximately $16 to $20 per square yard for good-quality nylon carpeting.

2. Carpeting is especially useful for the floors in an older building being renovated. Irregular, worn floors can usually be carpeted with minimal preparation, compared with the complete resurfacing needed before sheet vinyl or vinyl asbestos tile can be laid.

3. Be sure to have padding installed under your carpets. It adds to their bounce and their sound-reducing quality, although sound reduction seems related more to the carpet's pile height than to any other factor.

4. Don't order nylon carpeting for any area where strong acids, phenol, or formic acid will be used. Although nylon is impervious to most solvents, these three will dissolve it.

5. When your carpeting is ordered, be sure that the dealer knows that you want him to leave any usable remnants for future use in patching damage to the carpet.

RESILIENT FLOOR COVERINGS

The two materials in this category that are likely to interest you are the vinyl-asbestos tiles and the sheet vinyls. Of these, sheet vinyl is much more popular because of the smaller number of seams that can trap dirt or toxic substances, such as mercury.

Look for a *wear layer* (surface thickness) with a high content of vinyl and for a thick gauge (the overall thickness of vinyl plus backing). Suitable wear layers can range from .020 to .050 inch with a gauge of .090 to .100 inch.

All our treatment-room floors are covered with sheet vinyl with a separate vinyl cove base. This base is cemented to the wall and the floor. Its curved lower edge helps to prevent dirt collection.

Some special techniques of laying sheet vinyl are available. A process called *seam sealing* closes the crevices between adjacent widths of floor covering. Another process involves running the vinyl up the wall for a few inches to replace the separate plastic base or wooden baseboard. Producing this *cove* or *radius* completely eliminates the dirt collecting crack where the wall meets the floor. Both of these processes add to the cost of your floor. You'll have to decide for yourself if they're worth the price.

If you want to use sheet vinyl (1980 price: $10 to $14 per square yard installed), first find a reputable dealer (or include the flooring in your contract with the builder). Most of the major flooring manufacturers produce commercial vinyls suitable for your office. Select a color that won't fade in sunlight. (Ours is made up of different shades of beige and tan.) Also, if the vinyl has a resilient backing it will be more comfortable to walk on.

The preparation of the subfloor surface is much more critical for resilient flooring than for carpeting. It must be smooth and level. If it isn't, the vinyl will look bumpy, and the seams will open. In a new building, this shouldn't be a problem if the construction is correct. In an older building being renovated, however, it may be necessary first to put down a new surface of plywood or hardboard called an *underlayment*, if you want the sheet vinyl to be durable and attractive.

We learned this the hard way. The staff room in our office is located in the old part of the building. Its hardwood floors appeared only slightly irregular, so we decided against covering them with plywood before having the vinyl laid. Now we find that a seam is gaping and the surface doesn't look smooth. We've had to nail down the edges of the open seam to prevent their projecting up and tripping someone. Fortunately, our treatment-room floors were properly prepared with smooth plywood before the vinyl was installed.

40
WALL COVERINGS AND WINDOW TREATMENTS

You have a wide variety of materials to choose from when you start thinking about wall coverings. If you've engaged an interior designer, you can expect him to offer suggestions, but you can start thinking now about each area in the office and how it's to be used:

☐ Is it subject to heavy usage, such as a hallway or lobby?

☐ In the lab, sterilizing area, and darkroom, will substances be used that are likely to stain or soil the wall surfaces?

☐ Are people likely to touch the wall frequently, as in the waiting room and lavatory?

☐ In your treatment rooms and private offices, will wall surfaces be seen but rarely touched?

Let's look at various materials and see if they're good choices for such areas:

Paint. Paint is inexpensive, compared to other substances, and labor costs are relatively low. For that reason, it's the wall covering most landlords offer. If your lease calls for redecorating, that's what you'll get, unless you can negotiate a credit with the landlord and have some other material used instead.

Paint's advantages include ease of touch-up, if a surface is stained or scratched, and fairly easy maintenance. Many paints stand up to repeated wiping, but few can take repeated scrubbing.

A major disadvantage of paint is that it needs a new application about every two to three years to maintain a good appearance.

Caution: Even if your office is to be painted now, you should plan ahead to possible future use of wallpaper or vinyl if you own the building and plan to be there for quite a few years. All newly built wallboard partitions should be primed—given a first coat—with the kind of primer that will later permit the release of wallpaper adhesive. Here's why: If a wall is painted without being properly primed, and if wallpaper or vinyl wall covering is later glued to the wall, when that paper or vinyl must be removed, it may pull away the surface paper on the gypsum wallboard, leaving an unpleasantly rough surface. So tell your painter to prepare the wall for paper. This won't interfere in any way with the subsequent coats of paint to be applied.

Stain. Doors and wood trim around doorways and windows, especially if they have an attractive grain, can be stained to any desired wood tone. It can be scratched, however, and touch-up with a matching putty stick is necessary. Also, stain is practical only when the trim is newly installed. Once it's been painted, you'll have to repaint it each time you redecorate.

Wallpaper. Although wallpaper is an attractive alternative to paint, it can be a problem when used on any office wall subject to abrasion. It tears easily and it won't take repeated scrubbing. We used four different paper photomurals on seldom-touched walls in four of our treatment rooms.

Vinyl wall covering. This is a highly practical solution to many of your wall-decorating needs because it has a tough surface that can be washed as often us necessary, and it comes in scores of attractive colors and designs. It requires skill to install it properly and it's several times more expensive than paint. However, it can last 10 years or more before it needs replacement.

On the negative side, vinyl can be difficult to repair if it tears, and some people seem to have an uncontrollable urge to pick at torn or lifted corners. For that reason, raised corners should be glued back immediately. For outside corners (exposed edges where two walls meet), clear plastic corner protectors may be used if the corner is subject to abrasion or lifting of the vinyl.

Most of our office walls are covered with vinyl. The vestibule and part of the waiting room have a solid beige that blends with a mottled beige vertical corduroy surface in the remainder of the waiting room (see Figure 41-1).

The vinyl used for the treatment rooms, business office, sterilizing alcove, darkroom, staff lounge, and part of the hallway is an off-white grasscloth texture that is easily patched. Its light color adds brightness to the work areas. Its random design rarely shows dirt (see Figure 42-1).

The lavatories each have different vinyl wall surfaces. The patients' lavatory is decorated with a bright pattern of brown, white, and beige plus a silvery mylar that makes the small room seem larger. The staff lavatory has a pattern of 19th-century Parisian magazine ads. The trim—the door and window frames—in each lavatory is painted to blend with the background color of the wall covering.

Our private office has two different vinyls. Most of the walls are covered with an irregularly textured, predominantly rust and beige material (see Figure 41-5), while one accent wall has a look of smooth, rich Moroccan leather.

You don't have to buy the top-line vinyls (more than $20 per roll) for your walls to be attractive. Most of ours were less than $10 per roll in 1977.

As I suggested earlier, remember that you are decorating your office, not your home. Except for your private office, select materials, colors, and patterns that will be pleasing and relaxing to your patients and your staff as well as to yourself. One friend told me of the orange, brown, and black vinyl in a jagged pattern with which he covered the wall in one of his treatment rooms. It so upset his patients that several refused to be treated in that room. Needless to say, he had to replace the vinyl.

Wood paneling. Wood is one of the oldest and best-liked materials for covering walls. Its colors and textures can add warmth, distinction, and variety to any area in your office. We used horizontal, random-width, random-length, prefinished, red oak paneling in two of our hallways (see Figure 24-1). It was suggested by our architect, and it was supplied in tongue-and-groove strips that were glued to the underlying wallboard and nailed to the studs.

Our doors are also oak (see Figure 57-3). They and the window and door trim were stained to blend with the hall paneling.

Windows. Will your windows require covering at times for privacy or to limit the amount of outside light admitted? If so, you'll have to consider shades, blinds, drapes, or curtains alone or in combination. There are so many varieties of these that you'd better consult with your designer before deciding on one.

In your own building, you'll have more choices in your window treatments because you'll be able to select the windows themselves. In our new wing, we installed windows with thin venetian blinds between the inner and outer panes of glass (see Figure 41-5). These window/blind combinations are attractive, functional, and practically never need dusting or maintenance.

The windows in our waiting room don't need covering. Those that face the street are screened by tall evergreen shrubs planted by the previous owner. The other windows, in a bay, are decorated by hanging basket plants, but they don't need covering for privacy (see Figure 41-1).

41
FURNITURE

Long before the plans for your new office are finished, you should give serious thought to its furnishing. The earlier you order furniture, the better, because of the long delivery times involved. The right choice of furniture can add greatly to your patients' comfort and to your staff's morale.

Furniture can reflect so many images and moods that I won't attempt to discuss them. This is a matter for you and your designer to decide. Your choices will involve furniture period, scale, color, form, and texture. They should be chosen as carefully as everything else about your office.

We'll consider furniture in three broad categories—for patients, for your staff, and your own private office furniture.

Before you make any final choices, prepare cutouts to scale and see how they fit on your floor plan.

PATIENTS' FURNITURE

Unless your practice is one in which only one age group is treated, you should have several types of seating in your waiting room.

Older people, heavy people, and pregnant women find it difficult to get up from a soft low chair or sofa. For them, a firm straight chair at least 16 inches high with padded armrests is best. Chair arms should be about seven to eight and one-half inches above the seat. Individual armchairs should be at least 20 inches wide between the arms. Side chairs should be about 20 inches wide. Both should be 22 to 24 inches deep (front to back).

Young and middle-aged adults may enjoy a soft chair or sofa to relax in. Children, especially very young children, should have low chairs or a bench that permits them to sit with their feet reaching the floor. Consider, also, a children's alcove with appropriate chairs and playthings. Figure 41-1 shows the seating in our reception room.

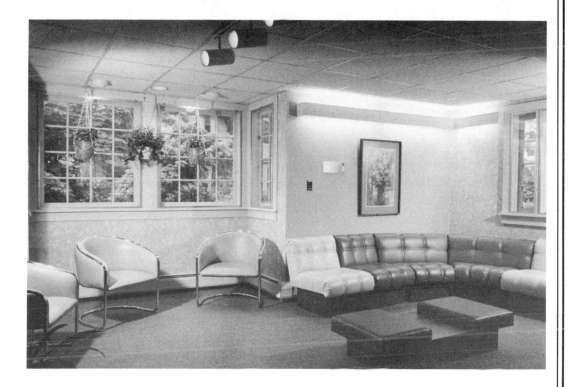

Figure 41-1. Reception room. Three types of seating are shown: firm barrel chairs, sectional corner sofa, and low bench. Sofa and bench have solid bases to minimize cleaning problems under them. Bench is used by young children. Lighting is by indirect *light cove* above sofa and coat rack (see Figure 57-3), and by individual *eyeball* and *highhat* fixtures above barrel chairs. Spotlights on ceiling track in foreground illuminate needlepoint tapestry and fireplace at left (see Figure 57-2). Hanging basket plants in bay window help to bring the outside greenery into the room. Beige vinyl wall-covering behind painting (and around fireplace) has a suede finish. Vinyl used elsewhere in room is a vertical corduroy in shades of beige (see Figures 57-2, 57-4D). Note rounded shapes of furniture and absence of jagged forms.

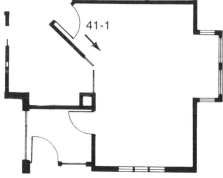

Most people will not choose to sit on a sofa close to a stranger. Instead, they'll look for a single chair. If you use a sofa, make it wide enough so that your patients won't be squeezed together. Place your reception-room chairs side by side or at angles to one another. You can avoid a clinic look by arranging the seating in clusters. But don't position chairs directly opposite each other. This forces their occupants into direct eye contact, which makes many people feel uncomfortable.

Although the style of the seating depends on the overall period and atmosphere in the room, you should give some thought to the lower part of the chairs or sofas. If you select a large number of individual chairs, each standing on its own four legs, you'll find that your waiting room appears to be a forest of chair legs that appear unattractive and make cleaning difficult. One satisfactory alternative is the use of modular seating; several individual seats are mounted on a single base that may be solid—thereby avoiding the need for frequent cleaning underneath—or with only a few legs. Sofas, too, can be bought or built with a solid piece of wood, metal, or plastic blocking off the open area under them. Floor cleaning is simplified, and you won't have patients or staff crawling around to retrieve balls, pens, or other items that have fallen and rolled under the sofa.

Any fabrics chosen should be those that repel dirt and are easy to clean. We've found that the substance that causes the most difficult stains is ballpoint pen ink. It's virtually impossible to remove from vinyl, and it causes problems with other fabrics as well.

BUSINESS-OFFICE FURNITURE

The chairs and desks you provide for your secretarial and business staff should be based on function. You want maximum efficiency combined with comfort.

Chairs. Your business-office assistants are likely to spend at least six or seven hours a day at their desks. Buy them the most comfortable chairs you can find. You'll be more than repaid by the boost it will give to morale.

Secretaries' chairs should be about 18 inches wide and 19 inches deep. Each should have four or five adjusting devices available for varying seat height, backrest height and position, backrest angle to seat, and backrest tension. It's important that you and your secretary know how to work these for her optimum comfort. If the chair doesn't come with printed instructions—and many don't—insist that the dealer show you how the adjustments are made. Write down the instructions if they're at all complicated. Tape them to the underside of the seat. Several years from now, when a new person occupies that chair, someone built differently from your present secretary, those written notes may prevent some head scratching and jammed fingers.

There is no law that requires a secretary or anyone else to use a secretary's chair. Those chairs are designed primarily for typists. If you have a staff member who works at a desk but does little or no typing, that person might like a swivel-type chair with arms.

Desks and countertops. We found that the most effective and least expensive way to create the proper desk and drawer space for our business office was to rely on ready-made metal drawer and file cabinet pedestals and custom-made countertops. Metal desk pedestals come in many different colors, drawer or cabinet combinations, and sizes.

Our cabinetmaker built the countertops to our design, supplied the pedestals, and later assembled them in our office (Figure 41-2, 41-3).

We decided on the size of desks and the drawer arrangements by listing the items—and their sizes—that would be used on and in the desk. For example, our appointments secretary needed space on her desk for these articles:

☐ appointment book (when open): 34" × 14";
☐ desk telephone: 10" × 8";

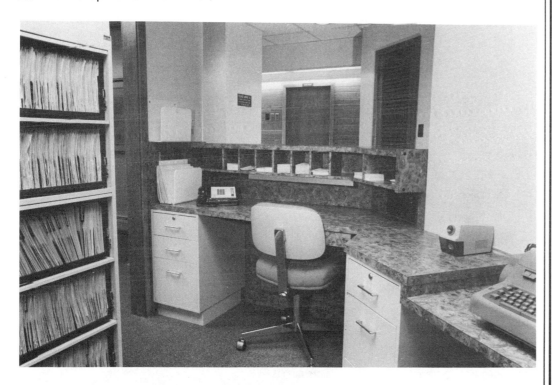

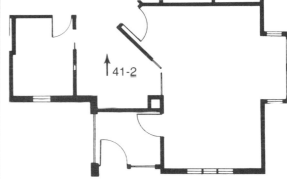

Figure 41-2. Appointment secretary's work area. Wrap-around desk is custom-built plastic laminate countertop with separate metal drawer pedestals. White plastic chart racks hold loose charts. Pigeon holes provide space for appointment cards, other forms. Note three-inch drop in counter height for typewriter. Secretary's chair has carpet casters, four-way adjustments. Strip fluorescent lamp (turned off) under pigeon holes gives added light to work area. For desk dimensions, see text. Louver door (right, rear) is to staff coat closet.

Figure 41-3. Business office as seen by patient standing at counter looking past appointment secretary's desk. Desk at left rear is used by insurance secretary who has view of reception room. Glass panel above her desk has opening for discussing insurance problems with patients. Counter at rear has telephone answering machine at left, postage scale and meter at right. Clear area of counter is used for chart assembly. Slots below answering machine hold groups of charts. Narrow window above counter gives secretaries view of entry vestibule. Patient records are kept in pull-out lateral file cabinets. Over-file cabinets with sliding doors at top right provide storage for office supplies. Location of typewriter permits its use by either secretary or by a third person. Adjacent bookkeeper's office has copying machine, printing calculator, second electric typewriter, and fireproof filing cabinet.

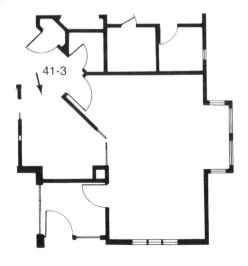

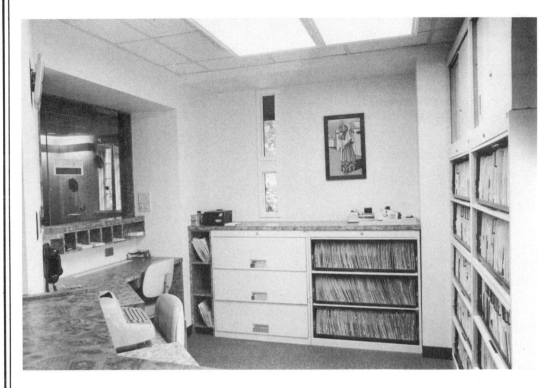

☐ pencil cup: 3″ diameter; and

☐ small rotary file of frequently used phone numbers: 3½″ × 3½″.

To accommodate these, we provided a desk top 64″ wide by 22″ deep. It gives her the space she needs for these items plus a little extra elbow room (see Figure 41-2).

If you use this approach, be careful about the front-to-back depth of such a desk. If this dimension is too shallow (less than 20 inches), the secretary will have inadequate space for working; if it is much more than 26 inches and there is a counter in front of the desk, your secretary will have an uncomfortably long reach to hand an appointment card to or accept a payment from a patient, especially if one of them has short arms.

Our secretary uses many small cards and forms. We had a series of pigeon-holes to fit these built under the countertop in front of the desk.

Drawers were needed for a removable box of 5½″ × 8½″ ledger cards, for filing 3½″ × 6″ cards, and for miscellaneous materials. The drawer pedestals each have two 5¾″ H × 13½″ W box drawers and one 11¼″ H × 13½″ W letter-size file drawer. The front-to-back depth of each drawer pedestal depends on the depth of the desk top above it.

We used the same approach for planning counter space for photocopying, for typing, and for work stations for our Insurance secretary and bookkeeper. By providing a form adapted to each area's function, we created an efficient business-office arrangement at minimal cost.

The desk and counter dimensions we arrived at, and that are working well in actual use, are:

☐ desk heights: 29½″;
☐ desk tops:
    appointments: 64″ × 22″
    insurance: 62″ × 20″, and
    bookkeeper: 71″ × 31″;
☐ typewriter countertops: 26½″ H × 28¼″ W × 20″ D;
☐ copying machine countertop: 26½″ H × 58″ W × 17½″ D;
☐ chart assembly countertop: 40″ H × 82″ W × 18½″ D; and
☐ patient appointments countertop: 44″ H × 75″ W × 9½″ D.

Before you plan your business-office furniture, read Chapter 45. Also, see Figures 41-4A and 4B to get ideas about the enclosure between your secretary and the reception room.

PRIVATE-OFFICE FURNITURE

The chair and desk you select for yourself in your private office depend partly on whether the room is to be used solely as a study or also as a consultation room. In either case, you'll want a chair that is comfortable and gives you adequate support. Here are a few guidelines:

1. You should be able to sit with your back against the backrest when your feet are flat on the floor. This means that if you're short, you shouldn't get a

Figures 41-4A and 4B. Secretary's glass partition. Fixed glass gives insurance secretary telephone privacy plus a full view of reception room, while opening, six inches wide, permits her to discuss patients' insurance questions away from appointments desk. Alternative is the frequently seen (but seldom moved) sliding window. Glass arrangement is shown on floor plan, Figure 19-4. Note signs and decals that make it obvious that the glass is there.

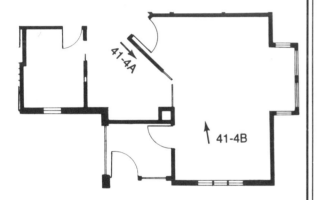

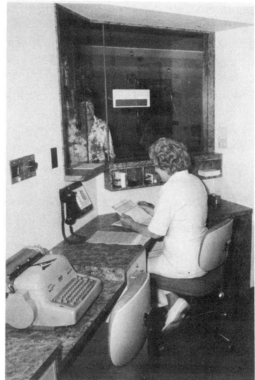

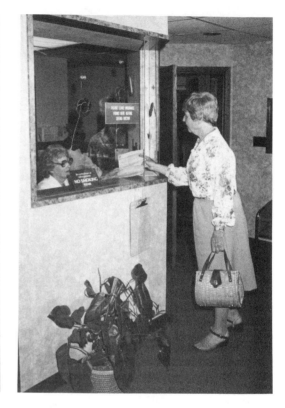

chair with too great a distance from the backrest to the front edge of the seat.

2. Several seat and backrest arrangements are available. The *swivel* type of executive chair has the seat and backrest at a fixed angle to each other, while a *posture* chair allows you to change the height of the backrest and its tension. Try each type before deciding. We found that our posture chairs were a good choice.

3. A cushioned seat with firm springs will support you more comfortably than a very soft one, if you use it for any length of time.

4. If your private-office carpet has a high pile, get a chair with oversize casters so you can easily move toward and away from your desk.

5. A seat-height adjustment is useful, even though you're the only one likely to use the chair. It permits adapting the height precisely to your needs.

6. If your chair will be positioned between your desk and a wall, allow about 40 to 48 inches between the wall and the edge of your desk for ease in going to and from the chair.

My partner and I use our private office only as a study and workroom. We wanted large desk tops, but we didn't want to spend the huge amounts that separate desks would cost. The architect's solution was to use the same type of custom countertop and prefab metal drawer pedestals as we used in the business office. In addition, we had a separate unit built to hold the charts or insurance forms that need our attention (Figure 41-5).

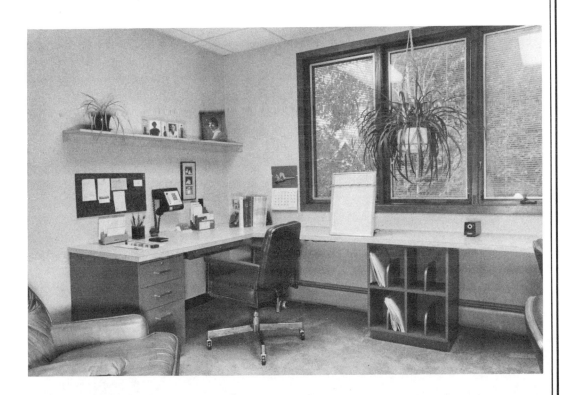

Figure 41-5. Private office. Spacious and inexpensive desks were created by combining metal drawer pedestals and pencil drawers with a plastic laminate countertop. Cabinetmaker also built chart rack, under window, for records needing doctors' attention. Countertop continues around to right to form two additional desks. Windows are casement type, with venetian blinds between inner and outer panes of glass. Posture chair has separately adjustable seat and back and extra large casters for easy rolling on thick, gold-colored, high-pile nylon carpet. Chair seat is fabric covered, which prevents occupant from sliding, while the arm rests and back are covered with vinyl, allowing freedom of movement of the upper body. Club chair in left foreground is a recliner.

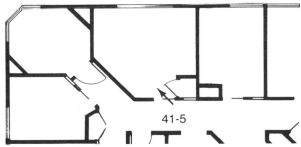

41-5

If you'll use your private office as a consultation room, you may want a handsome, impressive, wood desk. But don't assume that this is your only choice. You can still have a desk made the way we did. The sides that face the patient can have a layer of plastic laminate in the same wood grain finish as the top. The drawer pedestals, which you see but the patient doesn't, can be the ready-made inexpensive metal units.

For relaxation in our private office, we have a comfortable armchair that converts to a recliner by pulling a lever. It's great for those occasional few minutes between patients when one of us wants to stretch out.

42
CABINETS
AND BUILT-INS

Cabinets for your treatment rooms, lab, and sterilizing area are likely to be a major expense—possibly $1,500 or more per treatment room, for example. You'll avoid overspending if you understand how and by whom they are built and installed, and how you should go about planning them.

Fixed cabinets consist of one or more drawer units, sink units, or storage units that either rest on the floor (known as *base* cabinets) or are suspended on the wall (*wall-hung* cabinets). All visible sides of these units are covered by a plastic laminate. A separately built countertop is attached to the top of the base cabinets to provide a work surface (see Figure 42-1). Let's consider each of these components separately:

Drawer units. Drawers are the most expensive and difficult parts of the entire cabinet to build. For this reason, some cabinet manufacturers use prefabricated drawer shells in a limited number of sizes. Frequently used sizes are 3-, 6-, and 9-inch heights, 18- and 24-inch widths, and 12-, 18-, and 24-inch depths. Note, however, that these are *nominal* dimensions. The actual amount of open space within each drawer may be less or more. The only way to find out if a particular item will fit into a drawer is either to try it or to ask the manufacturer for the *clear, inside dimensions* of the drawer. We discuss below how to plan your drawer cabinets.

Sink units are designed to hide the underside of a built-in sink and its plumbing lines. They also provide storage space under the sink. Access is usually by doors, and often a swinging laundry door is also provided. The sink cabinet's dimensions will be determined by your sink size and by the height and depth of your countertop.

Storage units are made with a variety of fixed, adjustable, and/or sliding shelves, and they can be fitted with electrical and/or plumbing lines for installation of specific equipment. If dental treatment room plans call for side or rear delivery of air-driven handpieces, be sure that the projection of the equipment from the open cabinets won't interfere with the movement of patients or staff in the room.

Countertops are usually about 1¼ to 1½ inches thick, and they're covered with laminate on all visible surfaces. They rest on base cabinets (drawer, sink, and/or storage), and they can also extend over open space to provide extra work surface (see Figure 42-1).

Wall-hung units above the counter are often used to store prearranged trays of instruments for different procedures. They can be installed in each treatment room or in one central supply area (see Figure 42-2).

DESIGNING YOUR CABINETS

The following sequence of steps worked well for us:

1. Divide all the instruments and supplies that are to be used in each room into two groups:

☐ those that must be present in each room at all times, either separately or as part of prearranged sets, and

☐ those that are to be kept in a central supply area for delivery to the treatment room as needed.

For each group, list quantities of single items needed or the number of prearranged trays that you intend to have in each room.

2. Decide on the height and the front-to-back depth of your countertops. These are important because the height is related directly to your comfort while working and it may limit the number of drawers in your drawer cabinets. The depth will determine the capacity of your drawers.

If you work from a seated position, you'll want counters from 24 to 33 inches high. Ours are 33 inches. If you need access to the countertop primarily while standing, consider heights of 34 to 38 inches. The height you choose should depend at least in part on your height and arm length. If the work surface in question is to be used primarily by a seated assistant, a suitable height is about 29 to 30 inches. If she'll work from a standing position, 36 inches is best, since most women are accustomed to this height at their kitchen counters.

3. Calculate the vertical space available for drawers. This is the distance between the underside of the countertop and the top of the *toe space*. This space is usually about four inches high and is built into all base cabinets.

Since, as we already mentioned, drawers often come in 3-, 6-, and 9-inch nominal heights, figure out what combination of sizes will fit in the space available to you. The arrangement you select should be based on your list of instruments and the supplies that are to be kept in the drawers. These quantities should also permit you to calculate the drawer widths needed, frequently 18 or 24 inches.

If the vertical space available for drawers under the counter makes it apparent that you'll have insufficient drawer space, consider one or more of these alternatives:

☐ a second drawer cabinet;

☐ storage cabinet(s) above the counter using shelves instead of drawers;

☐ increased use of a central supply area; or

☐ a mobile cabinet with additional drawer space.

The front-to-back depth of your drawers will be limited by the size of the counter. Since most treatment-room counters are 12 or 18 inches deep, this will be the nominal depth of the drawers. But remember that the critical dimensions will be those of clear inside space.

4. Decide on the size of the sink(s) to be built into the countertops. Ours are 15½ inches wide by nine and one-half inches front to back. We find this size comfortable. The minimum width of the sink cabinet will be determined by the sink size, but it can be larger if you want more storage space under the sink.

If you intend to use a pedal-operated faucet for your sink, be sure to tell this to the cabinetmaker. He'll have to provide a cutout in the toe-space wall to permit the pedals to come through; he should also make a large trap door in the floor of the sink cabinet so the plumber can have access to the pedal-activated valves.

5. Design storage cabinets for special equipment based on the electric and/or plumbing needs and the size of the items. If a sliding shelf or some other device will be used to deliver the instruments closer to you, decide how much forward extension will be needed.

Figure 42-1. Treatment-room cabinet. Countertop (33 inches high) with attached backsplash is installed over separate drawer and sink pedestal units. Drawer pedestal is angled away from wall for easier access to drawers. Gap between this unit and wall is filled by triangular extension of backsplash (below cup dispenser). Open area below counter provides space for waste can and, when not in use, for operating stool. Sink has foot controls. Switch above and to right of phone is music-system volume control. Note toe space at base of drawer pedestal.

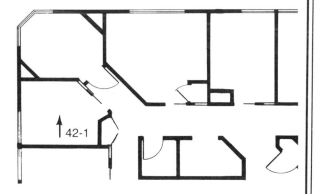

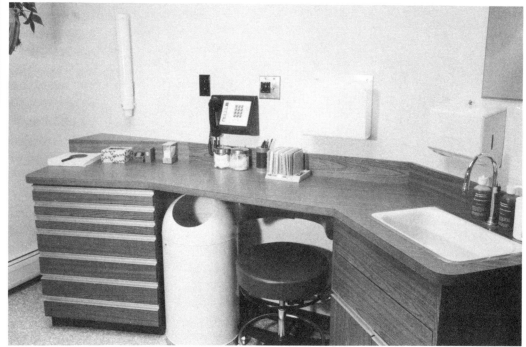

6. Plan the location of the various base cabinets in relation to your usual working positions, taking into account the frequency with which you and/or your assistant will need access to each. The base cabinets need not be right next to each other. The countertop can bridge any gaps, as shown in Figure 42-1.

7. Plan to have the corners of the countertop rounded where they jut into the room. A square corner of laminate can cause a painful hip or thigh injury to anyone who bumps into it.

8. Select colors for the plastic laminate to be used for the countertop and for the base cabinets. Since they're built separately, they don't have to be the same. Our treatment rooms contain some base cabinets with wood grains and some with solid colors. Our countertops are wood grains, solid colors, or butcher-block design. Choose plastic with a matte finish to minimize glare.

9. Finally, keep in mind these points:

☐ For maximum efficiency, plan to have identical cabinets and cabinet contents in every treatment room.

☐ You may be able to omit base cabinets entirely by using wall-hung units covered by a countertop if your storage needs are small. This will give a small room a more open feeling.

☐ Insist on up-and-down adjustable shelving in *all* storage cabinets; the size of items stored may change with time (Figure 42-2).

☐ Design lab or sterilizing-area cabinets and counters, using the same approach as outlined above: First analyze your needs, then decide on how much and what kind of built-in space is needed (Figure 42-3A, 3B).

☐ If you're considering a *casework* wall, a complete wall of built-ins, get professional design help.

☐ Lazy-Susan pivoting shelves are often not worth their extra cost because the space behind and alongside them is unusable.

☐ Sturdy hardware is important. You need substantial drawer and door pulls, hinges that permit opening a cabinet door 180° or even 270°, strong shelf supports, and full-extension drawer slides that permit access to the rearmost part of a drawer.

For the neatest professional-looking job, the installer should *scribe* (fit) the countertop in the room where it is to be installed rather than attempting to construct it completely from plans. Any irregularities in wall construction can result in gaps between the countertop and the wall if this scribing is not done. A good cabinetmaker will bring the countertops to your office after the spackling is completed, scribe them, and then take them back to his shop to complete the job.

Mobile cabinets are a specialized area of the cabinet field. You can often use a stock model or have one modified for your purposes rather than designing a completely custom cabinet. Since there is such a wide variety, I don't propose to discuss them in detail. However, the principles listed above work equally well here. Let function dictate form.

Durable hardware is especially vital on these cabinets. Casters must be large enough to roll freely on even a carpeted treatment-room floor.

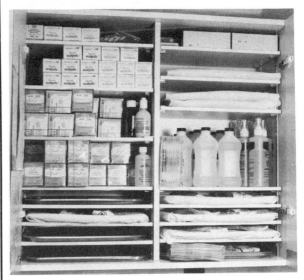

Figure 42-2. Wall cabinet in sterilization area. Adjustable shelf supports permit arranging shelves at different heights. Cabinet dimensions: $31\frac{1}{2}$"W × 28"H × 12"D.

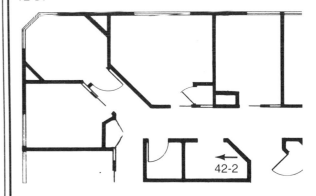

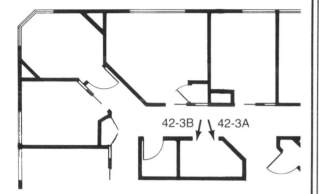

Figures 42-3A and 3B. Sterilization and central-supply alcove. Deep (10½ inches) stainless-steel sink permits soaking dirty instruments without their being seen by passing patients. Work space at counter (36 inches high) is ample for cleaning and bagging instruments prior to autoclaving and for assembling tray setups of sterilized instruments. Drawers and cabinets below counter plus wall cabinet provide storage for central-supply items. Note that wall cabinet does not extend up to ceiling. To avoid need for step stool, the highest inside shelf should be no more than about 75 inches high. Exhaust fan above wall cabinet keeps area free of steam and odors. Gray horizontal strip above shelf supplies extra outlets for ultrasonic cleaner, other accessories. Perforated steel rectangle high on wall above outlet strip is for call system's audible signal. Gray plate just below strip contains indicator light for annunciator system, informing assistant working here that front door has been opened. Floor is beige sheet vinyl, also used in treatment rooms, staff lounge, and darkroom.

If you're a physician, I suggest visiting one of the larger *dental*-supply houses if you haven't found a suitable mobile cabinet for your needs through a medical supplier. Recent innovations in methods of dental treatment, utilizing one or more chairside assistants, have led to new designs in these cabinets.

Recognize that your drawer needs in either a fixed or a mobile cabinet may conflict with the counter height you want. In such a case, you'll have to compromise either or both.

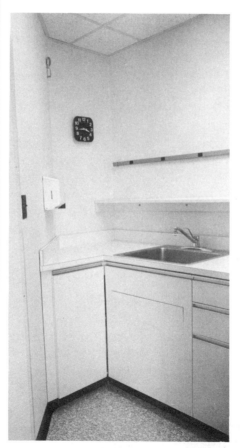

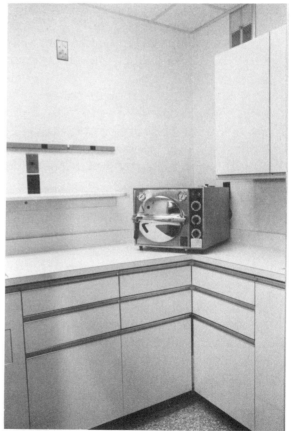

SOURCES OF CABINETS

There are three principal sources: Full-service equipment suppliers can obtain your cabinets from one of the major manufacturers or have the cabinets made for you by a local cabinetmaker. In either case, the dealer's service department will install the finished work and will honor the warranty.

Mail-order companies will send you literature showing their styles and sizes of cabinets. Since they may be hundreds or thousands of miles away, you'll have to find local workers to install the delivered pieces.

Local kitchen cabinetmakers sometimes make dental or medical cabinets as a sideline. Usually, they do the installations themselves. If you can find a good one, you'll probably save some money. The professional-equipment dealer must add his own overhead and profit to what he pays the cabinetmaker.

All our treatment-room cabinets and other built-ins were made by a cabinetmaking firm in a nearby town, which also supplied the metal drawer pedestals for our business and private offices. We selected them after speaking to several other doctors for whom they had worked.

Regardless of which course you choose, check the track record of the supplier carefully. This will be easier for local companies than for distant mail-order companies, but it's worthwhile for either Ask the previous customers: Was the company honorable in its dealings? Did it deliver on time? Was the price right? Were any of the cabinets delivered scratched or otherwise marred? Did the company correct the defects promptly? Was there a warranty? Was it honored? Has any of the hardware loosened or needed repair?

Prices of cabinets and countertops are difficult to discuss because of the many possible variations. The price of a drawer pedestal, for example, depends on its height, width, number of drawers, types of accessories, and shape of countertop. Laminate-covered countertops cost about $24 or more per linear foot (1980) for a 24-inch-deep top with a four-inch-high backsplash, but this price can be altered by the shape, edge form, and cutouts involved.

The best approach is to write down your needs as carefully and completely as possible before trying to shop for cabinets. Otherwise, you're likely to buy more or less than you need.

43

OFFICE
EQUIPMENT

In Chapter 19, I mentioned the need for allowing enough space in your business office for the various pieces of office equipment you're likely to buy. This chapter discusses the particular office equipment you're likely to need now or in the future.

Your primary concern, whether you're buying a typewriter, a copier, or a computer, is that the equipment works well and keeps on working. Ask the dealer the following questions about each piece of equipment. Then get the names of users from the dealer and ask them the same questions:

1. How long is the warranty? Who does the servicing, the dealer or the manufacturer? Some brands of telephone-answering machines, for example, aren't serviced by the retail stores that sell them. You have to ship them back to the manufacturer.

2. Does the machine jam or require frequent adjustment by staff?

3. How often does it require calling the dealer for service?

4. How soon after you call can you expect a repairman to arrive? Anything more than half a day is too long for an important piece of equipment.

5. Can most repairs be done in a short time—less than an hour—in your office and with parts carried by the repairman? It should be unnecessary, except in very rare instances, to take the equipment back to the dealer's shop. Will he provide you with a "loaner" when necessary, so that your office can continue to function while the repair is going on?

6. What doesn't it do too well? You're likely to get quite different responses to this one from the dealer and the users.

7. How long has this particular model been in use? If it's too short a time to develop a track record, you'd better be careful.

8. Another question you might ask the users is whether they know of anyone who's using this piece of equipment who *isn't* happy with it. Any names you get will be those the dealer is not likely to tell you about. Call them.

9. What part is likely to wear out first? In how long? How much will a replacement cost? How long after production of a particular model is stopped are replacement parts kept available?

10. If you were buying this item today, would you buy this brand?

Articles that describe the latest in office equipment are published occasionally in *Medical Economics.* If you have learned that *Medical Economics* has published an article that you'd like to see, you can write for a copy (Medical Economics, Oradell, New Jersey 07649), which they'll send at nominal cost.

The comments that follow are my own observations and not the result of any study.

TELEPHONE-ANSWERING MACHINES

These are available in two major types: *announce only* and *announce-record.* The first kind delivers a message to your caller, but it has no provision for his recording a message of his own. It's useful if your office will be closed for a long period and you want to direct the caller to another doctor. More likely, though, you'll want the second type, which allows the caller to record a message for you. As more of these devices are used, callers are becoming less reluctant to leave messages on them.

We're happy with a machine that uses removable tape cassettes for our announcement. On an old one, we had to record each new announcement daily. The new model permits us to use announcement tapes of varying lengths. More important, we've used the removable cassettes to provide our callers with specific information. We have announcement cassettes for each day of the week that the office is open. Before leaving each evening, our secretary plugs in the tape for the next office day. On most Friday nights, for example, she puts on the tape that says, "Our office is closed now until 9 o'clock Saturday morning." But if it's a holiday weekend and we won't be in again until Tuesday, she uses the tape that says, ". . . until 8 o'clock Tuesday morning."

For the sake of a patient in an emergency, we say on the announcement tape, "If it is very urgent that you reach me . . . please call my home." We don't give our home telephone numbers on the tape, but they are listed in the local directory. We feel that if it's important enough for the patient to reach us, he'll look it up. If it's a trivial problem, he or she is not likely to bother. In more than 12 years of using this approach, we've had very few patients abusing this availability of our home numbers.

FILE CABINETS

The two most popular types of file cabinets you'll probably consider for storing your records are the *vertical* and *lateral* cabinets. Let's consider each:

Vertical files have individual drawers, each of which is pulled out to reach the folders inside. Except for the fireproof kind, which I highly recommend for your most important records, I've found them much less practical than the lateral type.

Among the major disadvantages of vertical files are these:

☐ They extend 30 inches into the work area from the wall, compared with 18 inches for lateral files.

☐ They need more work space in front of them for the drawers to open than do lateral files. Drawers extend 27 inches, compared with 15 inches for lateral files.

☐ Most of them hold fewer charts per drawer than does a lateral file of the same size.

Lateral or shelf files are the type that display the edge of all the folders in each tier. Some have tiers that pull out, whereas others have stationary shelves. We've used the pull-out kind for 15 years (see Fig. 41-3), and we're convinced that they're the most practical type because of their capacity and the smaller aisle space needed in front of them. They hug the wall instead of projecting away from it. Two people can work side by side, pulling files from the same cabinet. This is impractical with vertical files.

Lateral files have one major hazard. They tend to have a high center of gravity, so they can tip easily. For this reason, they should be fastened to the wall behind them. The pull-out type is particularly susceptible to tipping if it's more than three drawers high. Although the mechanism is usually arranged to prevent more than one drawer being pulled out at the same time, this can sometimes be bypassed, allowing several drawers to come forward and increasing the tipping potential.

If you get lateral file cabinets, have them attached to the studs in the wall before they are filled with charts. Cabinets that are side by side should also be bolted to one another.

TYPEWRITERS

Unless the typing workload in your office is very light, you'd better get an electric machine. Most typists hate the manual models once they've used electrics.

If many of the letters sent out of your office are the same except for some minor additions, you may want to consider one of the *intelligent typewriters* or *word processors*. These are part typewriter and part computer. They store preset sentences or paragraphs that can be typed or altered on command. I've seen some of them in operation. They're impressive but they're also expensive: $5,000 and up.

COPIERS

Our office uses the copier for photocopy billing, for copies of insurance forms and correspondence, and for other miscellaneous jobs. We've found that a *coated paper* copier is adequate for our needs, even though the more expensive *plain paper* copiers produce a more attractive copy.

We looked for a photocopying machine that could take varying lengths of paper, including the 5½″ × 8½″ cards we use for patient ledgers. We also wanted a copier that was quiet, simple to use, permitted easy loading of paper and toner, did not jam frequently, and that produced a good-quality copy on a paper that later accepted handwritten notes in ballpoint ink (not all coated paper can be written on easily in ink).

We like the kind of copier in which the original lies on a glass plate rather than the kind with rollers that pull it into the machine. The latter permits faster feeding of the originals for billing, but we like the versatility of the first type, since we also copy from other materials.

There are many brands that are comparable in each price range. We chose our newest one because we had confidence in the dealer's reliability, after doing business with him for more than six years, and his speed of service.

COMPUTERS

For several years, we've heard how office computers will revolutionize paperwork procedures. That promise is nearing fulfillment as computers' prices fall and their capabilities multiply.

One major problem during the 1970s was that while the necessary hardware—the electronic equipment—was available, it was so expensive that it wasn't cost-effective for a small office. That is, its benefits weren't great enough to warrant paying the high price. With the development of the microprocessors, however, the price tags have been shrinking, as did those of pocket calculators a few years ago.

The second hurdle to be cleared was the lack of appropriate software, the programs needed by the machines. An explosion in software production is now going on for applications such as bookkeeping, billing, appointment control, and completion of insurance forms.

The computer field is changing so rapidly that I offer only some general suggestions about their possible use in your office. If there's any chance that you'll need a computer, be sure to provide sufficient space for it in your new business office. You'll need at least as much desk space as would be occupied by two large typewriters side by side. About half the space will be used by the terminal—a typewriter-like keyboard combined with a TV-like display screen—and the rest will be for the printer.

Before you shop for a computer, you'd better become well informed about their possibilities and problems. Read some books about computers in medical and dental applications. Subscribe to periodicals on the subject. If you talk to a computer salesperson with only some vague idea that you think you should computerize your office, you'll be a sitting duck. The salesperson will overwhelm you with all the wonders his machine can produce, but he won't tell you what it can't do or doesn't do well. The following "Questions to Ask Computer Vendors" is reprinted, with permission, from the October, 1979, issue of

Dental Economics. If you don't know what an acceptable answer should be to each question; you aren't ready to talk to a salesperson!

"1. How much does this system cost?

"2. Does this figure include programming as well as equipment?

"3. What components are included for this price?

"4. Are there additional charges for delivery, installation, etc.?

"5. How long has your company been in business?

"6. Is this system designed specifically for the dental [or the medical] office?

"7. Does this system have the capability to determine current account status at the time of treatment?

"8. How is treatment and fee information transmitted from the operatory to the computer?

"9. Does the patient receive a statement or receipt at the time of his visit? Is this computer-generated?

"10. How are data entered into the computer?

"11. How many active accounts can be stored in the computer's memory? Does the operator have to change disks to access certain accounts?

"12. Is a daysheet (daily journal page) generated? Does it show if any transactions have been changed or deleted during the day?

"13. Describe the system's audit trail. How can I check for errors or omissions?

"14. How are errors corrected?

"15. What kind of paper forms will I need? Will they require special printing? How difficult is it to change from one form to another?

"16. How are statements produced? How long should this take per 100? Are the forms separated, folded, and stuffed by hand?

"17. What is required to convert from my present system to the computer?

"18. How much training is provided for my office personnel? How much assistance can I expect from you during the conversion and start-up period?

"19. How is service handled on the hardware? How much does the service contract cost?

"20. How is service handled on the software? How much does the service contract cost?

"21. Can the software be updated as new programs are developed? Can it be modified to meet the specialized needs of my practice? How is this handled? What programming language is used?

"22. Can you provide names of other [doctors] who have purchased and are using your system?"

There's a strong possibility that the system the salesperson tries to sell you will be so new that it hasn't developed a track record. Ask when the first one was delivered and get the names of offices where it's been in use for six months or more. If there are none, look for another system. If there are satisfied users you can call, find out if the tasks done by their computers are the same as the ones you'll need. Visit at least two offices where *that system* is in use. Ask both the doctors and the assistants if they're satisfied with the system. Would they buy it again if they had the choice? If possible, take a knowledgeable consultant with you to help you evaluate the system.

The packaged programs being offered are usually based on the needs of the average office. If your office can use the software as written, that's fine. But if modifications, known as *customization* in the jargon of data processing, are needed, look out. Be skeptical if the salesperson assures you that "only a few minor changes" in the program will be needed. Ask if his company will accept full responsibility for those minor changes.

If the salesperson tells you that they'll send one of your assistants to their school for several days or weeks for training, the system is probably too sophisticated for your needs. What will happen if that person becomes ill or leaves?

If your office isn't well organized and smoothly running now, don't expect a computer to make it so. Switching to a computer will probably make things worse. The computer will highlight every inconsistency in your paperwork procedures. So if you're thinking of getting a computer, be prepared to scrutinize and possibly change some or many of the ways you're doing things. As a systems analyst put it, "Systemate before you automate!"

44
PROFESSIONAL EQUIPMENT

I'm willing to bet that if we asked 10 different doctors, "What kind and how much equipment will you buy for your new office?" we'd get 10 different answers, even if all were in the same field. And since equipment selection is so varied when different specialties are considered, I'll not attempt to make specific recommendations.

What I can offer, however, are a few guidelines that make sense, no matter what kind of practice you have:

1. Don't buy major items solely from a catalog or from a salesman's recommendation. They'll tell you only the positive features. See it and speak to one or more doctors who are using *that model.* The key questions are: What are the *bad* features of this equipment? Would you buy this model again if you had the chance? If not, why not?

2. Try to avoid being among the first to use any new model unless it's almost identical to an earlier, well-known version. The reason is obvious. You don't want to be the one who discovers the hidden bugs. Radical changes in equipment design may correct deficiencies of old equipment, but introduce unforeseen problems.

3. Even if you don't buy a particularly expensive piece of equipment now, do whatever messy work is needed to prepare the office for it at the time the rest of the construction is going on.

Examples are reinforcement of a wall to receive a heavy wall-hung item or lead-lining a future X-ray room. You won't want the dust and disturbance these jobs entail a few years from now when you buy the equipment. However, beware of going overboard in this direction. Have the preparatory work done only if it's *highly* likely that you'll get the equipment later.

4. Go first class! I can't emphasize this strongly enough. Penny-pinching is the wrong approach when frequently used equipment is being considered. Since the item may be used for 10 to 20 years or more, the difference between the best and the cheapest models becomes insignificant.

5. Remember discounts aren't everything! Your livelihood depends in part on the continued proper functioning of the equipment you buy. Your chief concern, then, should be finding the dealer who offers the best and promptest service, not the one who offers the lowest price. It's rare to find both attributes in the same dealer.

6. Before you discard a piece of usable and safe, but worn-looking, equipment, think about whether it can be refinished. Most equipment dealers can refer you to a refinisher or will have the job done for you. We had an X-ray machine in a color that was completely wrong for our new office decor. It was also somewhat battered from many years of use.

After having it checked by a radiation physicist who determined that it met all radiation safety requirements, we sent it off to a refinisher. When it was returned shortly after we moved into our new office, it looked like a new machine. The cost? $90 plus $45 for shipping both ways. The cost of a new machine was about $3,000.

Let me offer a few cautions, however, before you decide to keep and to refinish all your old equipment. Sometimes the cost of refinishing or reupholstering an examining chair or table just isn't worth it. And keeping some old equipment only because you're trying to save money is poor economy. You may be locking yourself permanently into bad posture and work habits caused by badly designed equipment.

Another problem with old equipment is the difficulty in getting replacement parts. I've learned from equipment service people that some manufacturers will declare their models obsolete after 15 or 20 years and stop making parts for them.

7. Order your new equipment well in advance. Dealers' delivery estimates are often excessively optimistic. If the equipment comes from the manufacturer before you need it, most dealers will warehouse it for you until you are ready for it.

FOR DENTISTS ONLY

You've undoubtedly read and heard of the controversy surrounding different forms of air-driven equipment delivery systems: "side," "rear," and "over-the-patient." After looking at some of the literature on the subject, I've reached the conclusion that there isn't any one best system. Each has its benefits and drawbacks. The *a-dec* Company has a free brochure that can help you understand the features of each. Write to: *a-dec*, 2601 Crestview Drive, Newberg, Ore. 97132.

We've found that a chair-mounted post that supports the light, the swing-away cuspidor, and an over-the-patient delivery system works well for us. But remember that ours is a specialty—periodontics—not a general practice. We work four-handed and two-handed at different times. Your pattern of practice may be quite different. I haven't found any one dental chair markedly superior to the rest. Most of them have similar features and adjustments. As long as the chairback is thin, the headrest is comfortable, the seat can go low enough (15 inches or less from the floor), and the motors work reliably, I don't know of any brand that significantly outperforms its competitors.

45

YOUR STAFF AND THE NEW OFFICE

Your office staff members will have mixed feelings about the move to new quarters, even though they may not voice them. On the one hand, a newer, larger office is appealing, but the prospect of new routines and possibly new staff members may create anxiety. Your awareness of this and your sensitivity to it will help you to prevent problems. Here are some points to consider:

1. Every office has a "pecking order," a sort of informal hierarchy usually based on seniority. Each person has his or her own "turf" or personal work space. Be sure to take this into account when planning the new work stations. For example, with two secretaries of approximately equal seniority in your business office, try to arrange for each to have similarly sized desks, chairs, drawers, and lighting. If you are insensitive to such needs, you may see a drop in productivity due to envy. If such an arrangement is impossible, consider some other tangible or intangible status element to make up for it. If one worker deserves more status, make it apparent.

2. Let your staff know that you're considering their needs for privacy (for example, by a staff lavatory), for security (such as a special place for their coats and handbags), and for comfort (possibly by a staff lounge) in your planning.

3. Since the move will present an ideal time to change many of your office systems, such as billing, record-keeping, inventory control, or sterilization, your staff may be worried about coping with proposed changes. Let them know well in advance what you have in mind and get their opinions.

The final decisions, however, must be made by you. Tell them what is going to be done, but reassure them that they'll be adequately trained in advance.

4. Other items we have found helpful for maintaining high staff morale include a refrigerator and a hot plate for lunches and snacks and a bulletin board in the staff room for notices and for minutes of our monthly staff meetings (for the benefit of part-timers who were not present).

5. During construction, especially when it's nearing completion, encourage your staff members to visit the new office to familiarize themselves with the room arrangement and traffic flow.

VIII
COPING WITH CONSTRUC-
TION

46

CLEARING
AND EXCAVATION

The first stage in the construction of your building will be the clearing of the land of unwanted vegetation. If many trees must come down, the builder will probably call in a tree service company to fell, cut up, and dispose of them. Not all wood is equally good for fireplace burning, so if you're thinking of arranging a side deal for the splitting and delivery of the wood to your home, be sure it's a type that you'll want to use.

Some wooded sites have particularly fine trees or shrubs you think should be saved. But even though they're not located where the building or parking area will be placed, attempts to save them could be a waste of time and money.

The reason is that the grading of the soil necessary to provide proper drainage around your building may raise or lower the soil level enough to fatally disturb a shallow-rooted tree's root system. If your architect and builder agree that a tree or shrub can be saved, be sure the builder marks it clearly with a bright ribbon or some other means of identifying it for the excavator. If the tree is particularly desirable, call in a tree expert before excavation starts to advise how to save it.

The next step is usually the rough grading of the property and the removal of stumps and large rocks with a bulldozer or some other earth-moving equipment. The grading is called *cutting* and *filling*—the reduction of high spots and the filling in of low areas with soil. Depending on the original topography, it could be necessary to dispose of excess fill or to bring some in.

The builder or a surveyor will mark the outlines of the building, the driveway, and the parking area with stakes in the ground and, sometimes, with taut string connecting the stakes. Using these guides, the excavator will dig to the level where the *footings* (the deepest parts of the foundation) are to be placed. This depth will depend on the climate in your section of the country and on whether your building is to have a basement. If temperatures drop below freezing in the winter, the footings must be below the *frost line*, the deepest level to which the earth freezes.

You'll be concerned about three possible problems during the excavation: water, rock, and poor soil. If digging uncovers masses of rock that are too large to be lifted out by machine, the builder will have to blast or drill them to more manageable chunks—at your extra expense, of course. If it turns out that the soil isn't firm enough to support the building, piles or a different foundation design may be needed.

Water, in the form of an underground stream, can be even more trouble. You can't block water; you must divert it somehow. This can mean additional cost for excavation and installation of extra drainage lines to carry the water away from the building to a lower area—if one can be found.

Water, soil, and rock problems can be detected by a soil analysis or by borings before work begins, but, I'm told, surprises still occur.

At about this same time, trenches will be dug from the main excavation to the street for the installation of utility lines such as water, gas, sewer, and electricity. These, too, must be below the frost line.

Your first impression when you see the completed excavation may be, as mine was, "Someone made a mistake! This is too small." Yet if you measure off the distances and compare your figures with the plans, they'll be correct. One reason for this apparent "shrinkage" is that your view of the excavation has the sky as its ceiling. In contrast, the excavated area looks puny.

Your architect and the local building inspector may require that the builder stop work at this point until they can inspect the excavation and the condition of the soil at the bottom. This soil on which the building will rest must be undisturbed and dense enough to bear the building's massive weight.

47
FOUNDATIONS

The footings of your building will probably be made of concrete. The carpenters erect *forms*, open enclosures of wood or metal that hold the poured concrete until it hardens; then the forms are removed. Properly constructed footings are very important, because the entire weight of the building rests on them.

Once the footings have hardened, work can start on the foundation walls. Masonry is used for any portion of the walls that will be underground. Usually, it will be poured concrete or blocks bonded together with mortar. Pipes that will later be connected to utility lines pass through the foundation wall.

In parts of the country where the soil is always moist, it's important that these underground walls be made impervious to moisture. Otherwise, your basement or even the rest of your building could have a constant damp feeling. Various techniques are used for this waterproofing. They include layers of cement, tar-like substances, and other materials sprayed or troweled on the wall.

Underground water that might collect outside the foundation is drained away by perforated pipes called *drain tiles* or *footing drains*. These are often installed around the outside of the footings and are covered with gravel. Water enters the pipe through the perforations. Since the pipe is pitched, the water runs to a low point away from the building or to a storm sewer.

Once the foundation walls are finished and waterproofed, the earth-moving machines return to *backfill.* They push earth into place around the outside of the foundation walls and establish the rough soil level around the building.

Final grading of the soil and the paving of walks, driveways, and parking areas will generally be done later. Sometimes the crushed rock base and a first rough layer of blacktop are done early. The smooth finish blacktop coat is usually delayed until the building is completed so that it won't be damaged by the heavy trucks and machines used for construction.

A concrete slab usually forms the floor of the basement. Several inches of gravel are placed over the soil inside the foundation walls, a plastic sheet covers the gravel—to block ground moisture from coming through the slab into the building—and then the slab is poured.

If your building has no basement and the slab is to be the subfloor of your office, it can't be poured until all plumbing and other utility lines have been installed in their proper locations over the gravel. Since it'll be difficult to move these lines later, be sure they're done right the first time!

You, your architect, and your equipment supplier should meticulously check the placement of each pipe and electrical conduit against the working drawings. The exact identification, location, and direction of flow in each line should be drawn on your copy of the plans. Also, take photos of all of these pipes and cables from several viewpoints before the cement slab is poured. These precautions will be of enormous value if it's necessary to dig up and change the location of one of the lines in the future.

48
FRAMING: YOUR BUILDING STARTS TO GROW

Once the building is "out of the ground," work can start on the skeleton of the structure. This is an exciting time. In spite of your anxieties—and there will be plenty of details to worry about—each visit to the construction site will bring a new feeling of pride. The building grows almost magically as the plans and specs change from lines on paper to solid, visible reality. It's a sculpture you should take the time to enjoy.

There are many different techniques and materials used for *framing*, so I'm going to describe only the one that I'm most familiar with. We renovated an old house for our office, but the work also entailed the addition of a substantial new wing. This was conventional wood-frame construction.

If yours will be a fireproof building, the underlying structure of the walls and floors will be made of steel, concrete, and masonry rather than of wood as described here.

The first part of the frame construction is the building of the first floor. Beams are laid on edge to span the space over the basement from one foundation wall or intermediate support to the one opposite. Sheets of plywood nailed to these *floor joists* form a *deck* or *subfloor*.

The framework of the outside walls is built of vertical two-by-fours called *studs*, their centers 16 inches apart. Openings for doors and windows are provided as shown on the plans.

While some carpenters are putting up interior partitions, others will be building the second-floor deck if there is to be one, or erecting the framework of the roof. Next, sheets of plywood, called *sheathing*, are nailed to the outer surface of the studs forming the outside walls and the roof. Over the sheathing, black building paper or some other water-resistant substance is stapled. Later, the building's outer skin—siding, brick veneer, or other material—will be added. On the inner surface of the outside wall, batts of insulation will be stapled between the studs.

Framing is one phase of the construction process that usually moves rapidly, so rapidly that you're likely to start thinking that all those stories you heard about construction delays were exaggerated. They weren't. Things will soon slow down, as you'll see. The framing phase is the time when errors can be caught and corrected with the least loss of time.

Even with the best of intentions, a carpenter may misread the plans showing the placement of interior partitions. The result is a room the wrong size or a doorway or window opening in the wrong location. Go in on a weekend or some other time when the workmen aren't there and measure the room sizes, door openings, and other dimensions. If you find what seems to be an error, call the architect and let him instruct the builder to check it. This is a much better approach than to start yelling at the contractor or the carpenter yourself. A correction now will usually be a simple matter of moving some studs.

The following is a list of what to look for when you're in the framing stage:

☐ Are room layouts correct?

☐ Are room sizes correct?

☐ Check critical dimensions: Is space available for that special piece of equipment between a wall and a doorway, for example? Remember that the rooms will be at least one or two inches smaller in each dimension after wallboard and/or paneling are added.

☐ Are hallway widths correct?

☐ Are doorway widths correct?

☐ Is there reinforcement of walls in places where heavy wall-hung equipment is to be installed?

☐ Is there special wall construction for acoustic control?

☐ Is there sufficient space for pipes in walls?

49
ROUGH-INS AND INSULATION

As the framing is finished, the mechanical tradesmen can start their work. Plumbers, electricians, telephone people, alarm suppliers, and heating and air-conditioning installers *rough-in* the pipes, wires, tubing, and ducts that will later be hidden in your walls.

If your equipment supplier is on the job, he'll use an equipment template to mark on the studs or on the subfloor the exact locations where the plumbing and electrical lines must come through for later hook-up to your equipment. This is important, for the architect's drawings will show which utilities are needed in each room, but not precisely where. Try to be there when the final spotting of the equipment locations is done for the tradesmen. If this isn't possible, you should meet with the equipment dealer earlier at the site and decide together on the equipment placement. We found it helpful to make full-size paper templates of some critical pieces of equipment to help us decide on their exact locations. If you leave everything to the dealer, you're sure to have some unpleasant surprises much later.

The rough-in stage can take three or four weeks or more, especially if heating and air-conditioning ductwork is being installed. Dental offices are likely to need more time than medical suites at this stage because of the separate tubing for compressed air, central suction, and nitrous oxide-oxygen.

Before the walls can be closed and the pipes and wires hidden from view, rough-in work must usually be inspected by the local building inspector and/or the underwriters' (electrical) inspector.

Go into the unfinished office with your camera and electronic flash after the rough-ins are finished, but before the walls are closed. Take a picture of each wall that has piping or complicated wiring. Such photos can be valuable months or years later when you are thinking of changing a partition, putting in a new doorway, or installing some new equipment (see Figure 49-1). For a similar strategy, if your office is over a cement slab in a new building, see the last part of Chapter 47.

Before closing the walls, wall insulation will be installed in all outside walls and in interior partitions where it is needed to help your soundproofing.

If yours is a new building, you'll want to be sure that cracks and chinks in the outside walls are closed off. The places to look for them are around window frames and alongside any electrical boxes installed in the wall for outside fixtures. This isn't important for you, if your office is in a part of the country where cold weather is rare. But if you practice, as I do, where there is lots of blustery winter weather, you'll want your building to be as weathertight as possible both for comfort and for energy conservation.

Once the interior walls are closed, these openings are impossible to find without ripping off the wallboard. So walk through the building during daylight hours before the walls are closed, and you'll be able to see the gaps I'm talking about. If you're not certain that the builder will have them plugged, do it yourself with some spare bits of insulation or anything else that's available.

Trying to assign responsibility for this particular job is likely to be frustrating. The fit of the edge of the sheathing against the window frame, for example, is a carpenter's job; the cutouts for the exterior electrical boxes are done by the electricians; the insulation may be put in place by others, but none of these workers will be around months later when you discover drafts or cold wall surfaces in some rooms due to those small openings in the outside walls.

WHAT TO LOOK FOR

Plumbing:

   1. Are lines and valves for master water shut-off in the proper location?

   2. Are templates provided for all equipment?

   3. Are the lines in proper location in each room? Look for lines for hot and cold water, waste, compressed air, gas, central suction, nitrous oxide/oxygen. Have all lines been pressure tested for leaks?

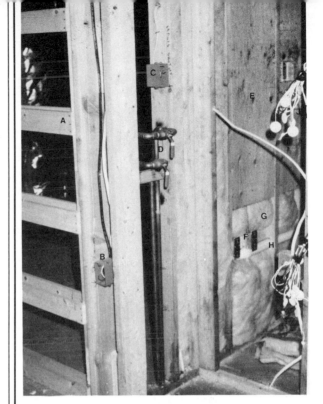

Figure 49-1. Closet, before wallboard installation. Pictures of office walls before they are covered with gypsum wallboard record locations of important pipes and wires and provide valuable information about construction. This photo shows:
A-frame for sliding door of room at left;
B-wires to duplex wall outlet;
C-master electric shut-off;
D-valves and pipes for master plumbing shut-off;
E-plywood reinforcement of partition to receive a wall-mounted X-ray machine in room at right;
F-outlet boxes for nitrous oxide/oxygen;
G-insulation in partition to aid sound control;
H-vent pipe from sink in room at left; and
J-collected and labeled low-voltage wires for several systems.
Such photos will prevent needless demolition if changes are needed in the future.

4. Do all the lines terminate in proper location in basement or utility room?

5. Does the plumber know heights for wall-hung fixtures?

6. Have any special venting requirements been explained *in writing* to the plumber? For instance, some central suction systems may require venting to the outside of the building.

7. Has provision been made for water filters, pressure reducers, mixing valves, other special equipment?

8. If you're going to have foot controls for your treatment-room sinks, have the lines to the foot-control valves been placed right or left of the sink's center?

9. Have cleanout plugs been placed in drain lines?

Heating, ventilating, and air conditioning (HVAC):

1. Have ducts for forced air heat and/or air conditioning been installed in each room?

2. Are there pipes for the baseboard hot-water system in each room?

3. Have heating lines been provided for hallways, basements, and other in-frequently used areas?

4. Are thermostats placed where they won't be affected by drafts or sunlight?

5. Have all chinks in the outside walls been plugged?

Electrical

Future wall outlets, electrical fixtures, and switches are seen at this stage as open metal or plastic boxes with wires in them.

1. Are wall outlets correctly located around each room and at the indicated height above the floor? Are they horizontal or vertical as desired? Are they straight, not askew?

2. Are special circuits properly located?

3. Are wall switches properly located and at desired height?

4. Are light-fixture boxes properly placed? Is there the right number of them?

Low-voltage electrical systems:

The wires for these systems usually don't terminate in boxes as do the lines that carry higher voltages. Instead, a low-voltage cable exits from the wall through a metal plate nailed to a stud. This plate, called a *plaster ring*, has a rectangular or square opening in it. Its presence will tell the wallboard installer to cut an opening in the wallboard at that location for the wires.

1. Are telephone outlets at the proper locations and height? Is the phone junction box panel in the proper location (usually in basement or utility room)?

2. Are intercom wires properly placed?

3. Are the wires for signaling systems in proper locations, including lines for buzzers, lights, switches?

4. Is the music system wiring all in place, including wires to each speaker and each room's volume control?

5. Are burglar- and fire-alarm cables installed at all necessary locations?

6. Are wires for other special systems installed?

7. At every location where switches, signal lights, and/or outlets are side by side, are the boxes or plaster rings installed at precisely the same height? If not, the finished installation is going to look sloppy.

8. Are all plaster rings straight? If not, the overlying wall plates that screw to them will also be angled.

50
WALLS
AND
CEILINGS

The gypsum wallboard used for the walls in your office comes in sheets four feet wide and eight to 12 feet long. It's usually one-half or five-eighths of an inch thick. As it's nailed to the studs, each nail is driven just slightly below the outer surface of the wallboard to form a dimple.

These nail depressions and the seams where one slab of wallboard meets its neighbor are filled with a joint compound, called spackle. The seams are covered with a special tape. The spackle shrinks as it dries, so several layers must be troweled on, a day or two apart.

The whole operation is a messy one, and you might as well stay away while it's going on. There's little you can do now, anyway.

Once the spackling is completed, however, you should look at and feel the smoothness of the walls. If the spackle is left rough or pitted in many areas, your painter or paperhanger will have a more difficult job later.

At about this time, the framework for the dropped ceiling will be installed. It will be suspended from the floor above or from the roof.

The ceiling squares or rectangles themselves may not be installed until later to avoid their being soiled by the work still to be done.

What to look for:

1. Are the joints and nail dimples filled and as smooth as the rest of the wall?
2. Are all corners neatly taped and spackled?
3. Is the ceiling framework symmetrical and level?

51
"FINISH" CARPENTRY AND MECHANICAL INSTALLATIONS

The finishing process in construction will drive you crazy if you don't know what to expect. It's the hardest to understand because what needs to be done seems like just a small group of little things that you think should take only a day or two. Unfortunately, even little things take time, especially if they are to be done well, and there are many more of them than you think.

Take doors, for example. Have you ever in your mind run through all the steps of a door's installation? Here's a quick rundown:

☐ The door opening is built with two-by-fours during framing.

☐ The door frame (sides and top) is cut to size and nailed in place. Sometimes a prefab metal frame is used instead.

☐ The recesses for hinges must be chiseled into the frame (in a prefab frame, the recesses are already there).

☐ The door is cut to fit the frame and is made short enough to clear your future floor covering.

☐ Recesses for hinges are chiseled or routed into the door.

☐ Hinges are screwed in place and door hung.

☐ The door stops and wood trim for both sides and top of door frame are cut, mitered, and nailed in place.

☐ The door and door frame are drilled for latch and knob installation.

☐ The latch and knobs are installed.

☐ The door is stained and varnished or painted.

All this is for just a simple interior door. Note that at least two or three different workmen will have worked on that door: a framing carpenter, a finishing carpenter (sometimes one carpenter does both), and a painter. If it's an outside door, you'll also need a locksmith and a weatherstripping specialist. These workers are not standing in line waiting to work on your door. Days or weeks go by while your job waits for a particular worker to arrive.

Now multiply this process by many doors, add sequences for the other parts of the office, add delays in deliveries, and you'll start to have an idea of why this stage in your office (and building) construction takes so long.

The finishing stage will have the greatest interest for you because the work done now will remain visible as long as you occupy the office. There will be a stronger temptation than before to scrutinize everything and to complain loudly as soon as an error is detected. But restrain yourself! If you've done your planning properly and you and your architect have watched the proceedings closely up to this point, most of the problems that arise now should be easy to correct.

As the finishing process continues, you'll spot things that need to be changed. Don't phone the architect or the builder every time you see something wrong, unless it's really a whopper. Instead, start a *punch list*. This term is used in the building trades for the list of specific details that must be done or corrected.

At intervals—approximately every seven to 10 days, say—call or send your list to the architect. He'll have a list of his own if he's been inspecting the job as he should. Let him be the one to tell the builder or the workers where and how to correct the errors.

Be positive and friendly in your conversations with the workmen if you visit the job while they're at work. Compliment them on work that's going well. Leave the critical comments to the architect and/or the contractor. Let them be the heavies. If the workmen think of Doc as a "good Joe," you're sure to get better work than if they consider you a nitpicking creep.

While the carpenters are working on trim, doors, and hardware, other tradesmen will also be busy. Electricians will be installing fixtures and wiring wall outlets and switches. Plumbers will attach toilets and sinks, except for sinks that will be mounted in cabinet countertops. Once the second layer of the subfloor is in (for wood floors there should be two), the heating people can connect base-board heating units. Air-conditioning systems can be hooked up, too.

Suddenly, your office will have light, heat or air conditioning, and power. It'll start to look like what you've been planning and dreaming about for months. Water will be turned on a little later, when all sinks and other plumbing fixtures are in.

WHAT TO LOOK FOR

Plumbing:

1. Are toilets and sinks securely fastened to floor or walls?
2. Are the compressor and suction systems connected?
3. Are nitrous oxide/oxygen outlets installed in treatment rooms?
4. Do hot and cold water lines work with adequate pressure?

Carpentry:

1. Do the trim pieces around doors and windows appear neatly cut and nailed? Are there any hammer dents?
2. Are the miter joints close fitting?
3. Do hinged doors swing freely and latch properly? Do sliding doors glide smoothly with little effort and without binding?
4. Do windows operate properly?
5. Is the hardware installation neat?
6. Are toilet-paper and paper-towel holders installed in the lavatories?
7. Are all plywood floors securely nailed? Are they smooth and level?

Electrical:

1. Are wall outlets neat and properly oriented horizontally or vertically?
2. Do the wall switches operate correct fixtures or outlets? Do the three- or four-way switches work as planned? If not, now is the time to have this type of mistake corrected—before walls are painted or papered.
3. Are all circuit breakers identified on the breaker panel?
4. Have all low-voltage systems—music, intercom, signaling, alarms—been tested, and do they operate properly?

52
CHANGE ORDERS

Any changes to the plans or specs that take place after the construction contract is signed are called *extras* or, more formally, *change orders.* A principal reason for having your plans and specs as complete as possible is the hard truth that change orders are expensive.

Every time you request an extra, you'll probably pay for it at full price plus labor plus overhead plus profit. Still, there are ways to keep these costs down.

The worst thing you can do when you think a change or addition is needed is to walk up to the workman or subcontractor on the job and tell him to do it. You'll then have to pay whatever the builder later decides to charge you, exorbitant or not.

The way to keep extras from getting out of hand is to have an inviolate rule agreed to by you and your partners that *no* changes are to be made without a written change order from the architect. (In emergency situations, the architect may give a spoken change order.) There are good reasons for this:

1. If you discuss the needed change with the architect first, he may be able to suggest other and possibly less expensive ways of doing the same thing. Changes that appear simple and uncomplicated to you may, if done as you ask, cause serious problems that you haven't even considered.

2. If an inquiry about the cost of a proposed extra comes from the architect, the builder knows that he'll be asked to justify any outlandish figures he quotes. A knowledgeable architect will be able to discuss choices of materials and methods and, in general, will be able to negotiate a more favorable price than you will. He may be able to arrange credits for some items that are less important in exchange for others that are suddenly needed.

3. Once the change order is in writing, there will be no future arguments about the price of an extra. Two people invariably have different memories of the same conversation. *Get it in writing!*

53
FINAL GRADING, PAVING, AND LANDSCAPING

The timing of this phase of construction often depends on the weather as much as on the contractor's work schedule. The earth-moving equipment will grade the land around your building to its final contours based on drainage needs and on your landscape design, if you have one. Walks, driveways, and parking areas will be marked out with stakes. Several inches of crushed rock or gravel will be spread to permit drainage under the hard top surface. Asphalt-paving material (blacktop) is spread and rolled smooth while it's hot. It's usually installed in two applications, a lower rough layer, which provides the bulk of the paving, and an upper finish coat.

Although the grading and paving can be done at almost any time after the building is "out of the ground"—when the foundation is completed—the landscape work will have to wait until the building is virtually completed and all the construction debris is carted off. Then your landscaper can rake the areas to be planted, and prepare the soil for lawns, plants, and/or trees.

Don't be in a hurry to get the planting done if it's the wrong season of the year. Far better to let the site appear barren for several months than to plant prematurely and risk the death of expensive shrubs and trees.

What to look for:

1. Has all debris been completely removed? Sometimes contractors attempt to dispose of construction debris by burying it on the property to avoid the cost of trucking it to a dump. The result is later settling of the soil, creating depressions in lawns or cracking of paved areas. Debris removal should include not just bulky items, but cleanup of beer cans, the remains of workmen's lunches, and assorted trash as well.

2. Does the paving look smooth and without depressions or cracks? These can collect rainwater that, in northern areas, may freeze in the winter.

3. Do plant materials look healthy and properly installed in their new homes? The nursery that supplies them should guarantee them—for both replacement and labor costs—through at least one full growing season.

IX
THE END IS IN SIGHT

54

PLANNING
THE MOVE

Here are some ideas that worked for us in the move to our new office:

1. Start planning three to four months in advance. That's when you should start going through drawers and closets, throwing out whatever you don't intend to take with you. You'll get a more realistic idea of what you have and how many cartons you'll need to carry it.

You have more than you think! Our 700-square-foot old office filled more than 60 cartons in addition to equipment, furniture, and packaged supplies.

2. Plan where each article of furniture and equipment is to go in the new office. Prepare a large tag—two by four inches with string attached—for each item. Print in large bold letters the name of the intended room. These tags will permit the movers or one of your staff to direct each article properly.

3. Hire the moving company early. If it's at all possible, find one with experience in moving professional equipment. An inexperienced mover may have problems with the weight distribution of some of your equipment, especially pedestal units, chairs, and examining tables. You won't appreciate a puddle of hydraulic oil spilled from a chairbase on your newly installed carpeting, and if a piece of equipment is dropped, you may not find out about the damage until a day or two later, after the mover has been paid. We found our mover through our equipment-supply company.

Long before moving day, have a moving company representative come to your office to look at what's to be moved. Get a flat price if you can, not an hourly cost, though flat rates may not be permitted for interstate moves. If he's a reputable, experienced mover, he can be pretty accurate.

The mover's visit can help you in a few other ways. Ask him:

☐ which instruments can be left in drawers and which ones must be removed.

Many hand instruments can be left in trays in drawers if you place towels over them to prevent their rattling around.

☐ if there are any fragile items his men will hesitate to move, such as the head of an X-ray machine. Most movers refuse to move living things, such as fish in an aquarium and live plants. You'll have to move those yourself.

☐ what kind of insurance is provided and what other coverages are available. To movers, damage is something that is visible. They may refuse to accept responsibility for internal mechanical harm to delicate equipment. Also, they'll usually be responsible only for items they pack themselves.

☐ which file cabinets must be emptied. Some four- or five-drawer files may be moved with the folders in them. A large fireproof file, however, weighs more than 600 pounds empty, and its contents should be removed.

☐ whether there will be problems getting oversize items out of the old building and into the new one.

☐ approximately how many cartons you'll need.

☐ how he expects to be paid. A mover referred to you by your supply company will almost certainly accept your personal or professional corporation check. But a mover to whom you are a stranger could demand cash or a certified check.

4. Discuss details of the move with your equipment company. You'll need their servicemen to disconnect and reconnect your old equipment and to install your newly purchased items. We moved three treatment rooms of equipment and newly equipped two others. To expedite the process, we arranged to have the new equipment installed during the week before we moved so that we could use it while the mechanics were hooking up the old chairs and units.

Again, try to get a flat fee for the equipment company's part in the move rather than an hourly figure. Their charge will include their servicemen's time, but will not cover parts replacement made necessary by the move. Equipment companies in my area charge about $30 to $35 an hour (1980) for a serviceman's time, and the flat amount we paid was based on this.

If you are paying on an hourly basis, you could find yourself hovering over the mechanic, resenting it every time he stops work for a coffee break or a moment's chat with one of your staff. That's why a flat fee is often better.

If any of your old equipment is to be refinished, arrange for it to be done in the quickest way. One of our X-ray machines, which was to be spray painted, was disconnected with the rest of the old equipment on moving day, taken to the refinisher by our equipment man, and then installed about 10 days later in the new office.

5. Decide how many cartons you'll need and what size. We found that cartons 24 inches long by 12 inches high by 12 inches wide were excellent. They held our letter-size patient-record folders neatly with minimal excess space on the sides, and they were much cheaper than cardboard transfer files. They were also a good size for almost all other items to be packed. You can get these or any other standard-size cartons from a wholesale paper distributor in your area. Look him up in the Yellow Pages well in advance. He may not have the size you want in stock, but he can get it. Order plenty. You'll need them.

The cartons are delivered knocked down. You set them up and seal the bottoms with tape, which the paper dealer can also supply. We found that two-inch-wide vinyl tape was excellent, and we bought a tool for applying it easily. We also used the tape for sealing the tops of the cartons after they were filled.

Use a felt-tip marking pen for identifying in large letters the contents of each box and its room destination.

6. Check with your insurance agent on your coverages before, during, and after the move.

7. Arrange for your new telephones to be installed several days before you move. That way, if anything is done incorrectly, there'll be time to rectify it before it interferes with your office operation. Be sure, however, that phone service at the old office is not cut off until moving day.

8. We found that there was minimal disruption of office routine by moving on a Monday. We used Saturday and Sunday to tear the old place apart and to pack and label everything.

9. Order the announcement of your move at least three months in advance. This will allow time for printing and for reprinting, if necessary. Murphy's Law—if anything can go wrong, it will—was at work in our case: Our first batch was printed incorrectly. It'll also give your staff enough time to address the envelops to all of your patients and professional colleagues.

There's no need to have the date of your move printed on the announcement. It'll be difficult to predict the exact date—or in some cases even the month—of your move. Since you won't mail them until a day or two before moving day, everyone who gets one will know that you are now in your new office. The date of your move is of no importance to patients once it has occurred. Those patients who have appointments just after the move should be called during the preceding week to reconfirm appointments and to tell them of the move in case the announcement is late in arriving.

We found it helpful to enclose a map with the announcement. This showed the location of the new office in relation to the old one. We drew the map with only the important streets, highways, and landmarks included. You don't have to be a trained artist or a draftsman to do this. Draw it in whatever large scale you find comfortable. Take it to a local printer and have him reduce it photographically to the size of your announcement. Our patients told us they found this very useful. As a result, we had only a few late arrivals because patients were lost.

All your announcements should be addressed, stuffed, sealed, stamped, and sorted by ZIP code a few days before you move. Sorting them will speed their movement through the post office and expedite delivery.

10. A few days before the move, send notices to all licensing agencies, professional organizations, suppliers, and insurance companies. Since periodicals need six to eight weeks to change an address, notify them earlier. And arrange at the post office for mail to be forwarded.

11. Block out at least two or three days in your appointment book for the period when you expect to move. If there are unexpected delays later, you can block out other time and move many of those patients into the first group of empty time slots.

12. Meet with your staff in the new office before moving day to acquaint them with placement of major items. Assign responsibilities for different parts of the office.

13. If your move is in winter and the new office is in a newly constructed building, be sure that arrangements have been made for snow removal and sand spreading.

14. If either your old or new office is in a commercial office building and your move is planned for a night or a weekend, be certain that the building will be open and the elevators operating when you need them.

15. If you'll be moving into a new building, be sure you get a certificate of occupancy before your moving date. The C.O. is the official permit that the local building inspector must issue before the building may be occupied. It verifies that the building has complied with the municipality's building codes and that it can be safely used.

You could be in for trouble with the local authorities or with your insurance carrier if you move in before a C.O. is obtained. In many situations, however, the building inspector may issue a temporary C.O., which permits use of the building while the last phases of construction are being completed.

16. If you have any special plants worth moving to your new office, here are a few suggestions: Since you'll have to do it yourself, be sure the plants are healthy and free of parasites. Spray them a few weeks before the move to be sure. Ask your florist for suggestions about pruning, repotting, and watering. Pruning is especially advisable for large plants, since they'll probably have to fit into a car's back seat. You can get special plant packing materials from the mover if you ask for them in advance.

17. You may want to take photos of your old office before you dismantle it for future comparison with the finished new office, for a record of how equipment and furniture were positioned, or just for sentimental reasons.

18. Finally, decide what to do with furniture pieces and office equipment that you won't be taking with you. Consider the possibility of giving them to staff members, donating them to a religious organization or charity, or contributing them to a vocational training school.

If you prepare carefully for the move, you'll find that the whole experience can be managed without the need for tranquilizers. Plan far enough ahead and you'll look back on the move later as only a minor nuisance in the transition to your delightful new office.

55
FINISHING THE WALLS, CEILINGS, AND FLOORS

Even though you're eager to get your new place decorated, don't let the painters start until the mechanical trades are finished and all their assorted garbage and dirt are removed. If you try to overlap the workmen too closely, you'll regret it. Dirty fingermarks on newly painted walls or sawdust in the air roughening your freshly painted or stained surfaces will mar these finishes.

This is the sequence in decorating that worked well for us:

☐ painting (including staining of natural wood surfaces and priming of walls to be covered with wallpaper or vinyl,

☐ paperhanging—installation of vinyl wallcovering,

☐ paneling—installation of prefinished panels,

☐ ceilings—installation of acoustic ceiling tiles in the previously hung grid, and

☐ floor covering. Carpeting and resilient flooring (vinyl or vinyl-asbestos) should be laid only after the mess of painting, papering, and/or paneling has been removed from the office.

Rooms that are to have resilient flooring should be checked by the flooring company ahead of time to be sure that the floor is smooth and level in all areas. If it isn't, the installer may refuse to lay the flooring until the subfloor is patched and leveled. His reason will be that the joints between sections of flooring will open later is placed over an improperly prepared floor.

Old walls, too, may require considerable patching to make them suitable for papering. Defects will be especially noticeable if light is directed down the wall from above.

Your burglar-alarm system may include the use of floor mat traps (under-the-carpet devices that trigger an alarm when that area is walked on). If so, the mats should be taped to the floor in the proper locations shortly before the carpet workmen come in. The wires from the mats must be arranged so that they won't be damaged by the strips of wood with nails protruding upward (called *tackless strips*), which the carpet installers will nail around the edges of the room. Be sure the alarm company is told when to do this. It should be no more than a day or two before the carpet is laid. If the mats are taped down too soon, they're likely to be damaged by other workers tripping on them or on the attached wires.

WHAT TO LOOK FOR

Painting:

1. Has all damage to wallboard been repaired? If there are many of these defects, you'll hear about it from the painters.

2. Have all nail holes—where nails were countersunk in door and window trim—been filled with putty?

3. Is the paint and/or stain smooth, even, without *drips*, *sags*, or *holidays?* (Drips and sags are self-explanatory; a holiday is an area missed by the painter's brush.)

4. Has the painter left small quantities of each type and color of paint for future touch-up purposes? Are the containers properly identified by the location where they were used?

Papering:

1. Was the paper or vinyl installed in the correct room? To avoid mixups, label each roll when it's delivered with the name of the room where it's to be hung, and put it in that room yourself.

2. Are there any air bubbles under the surface?

3. Are the seams straight, vertical, and without gaps?

4. Do patterns match from one sheet to the next?

5. Are the edges and corners glued down firmly?

6. Is the surface cleaned of all glue and debris?

Paneling:

1. Are the joints between panels tight?
2. Are the visible nail heads colored to match the paneling?
3. How are the cutouts for electrical outlets and wall switches? Holes in paneling must be small enough so that they'll be covered by the metal or plastic trim plates that are to be fastened over outlets and switches.
4. Are the top and bottom edges of plywood paneling covered by matching pieces of moulding?

Ceiling:

1. Do all ceiling tiles rest evenly in the framework?
2. Does the surface pattern in ceiling tiles lie in the right direction?
3. Are all tiles oriented the same way? You may never look up at the ceiling, but your patients—on an examining table or in a dental chair—will notice this.

Carpeting:

1. Are the seams tight where pieces are joined?
2. Are there bumps or gaps at walls?
3. Is the pattern oriented correctly?
4. Are transition strips where carpeting meets resilient flooring, usually at doorways, neatly installed?
5. Do the doors move freely above carpeting? Be careful not to have doors cut too short, or your efforts to soundproof a room may be defeated.

Resilient flooring:

1. Are there bumps or gaps at walls?
2. Are the seams tight where pieces join?
3. Is the pattern oriented correctly?
4. Is the vinyl cove base firmly cemented to wall and floor?

56

CABINET, FURNITURE, AND EQUIPMENT INSTALLATION

Once your floor coverings are in, your office will be ready for the delivery of all the things you ordered months before. Some suggestions:

1. Have someone present when deliveries are made, a person who knows what was ordered, in what colors, and where it is to go.

2. As the items arrive, your representative should inspect both the cartons and the article itself. If the carton and/or article is damaged, this should be noted on the receipt given to the deliverer.

3. Refuse to accept delivery of items that are obviously wrong or unusable. For example, one of our over-file storage cabinets was delivered with its sliding doors taped shut. When we removed the tape, we found that the final coat of paint had been sprayed on the cabinet *after* the tape was put on. Removal of the tape exposed a strip of the darker base coat of paint. It looked awful. We sent the cabinet back with the deliveryman.

4. If your purchase contract calls for the suppliers to unwrap the articles—of furniture, say—and remove the cartons and wrappings, be sure that they do it. You're going to have lots of garbage to be carted away. This tactic will help to keep it down. You'll be able to do it with some suppliers of furniture and office equipment, but usually only if it's agreed on in advance.

5. Ask for and save all operating and maintenance instructions, extra parts (be sure to label them), warranties, and copies of delivery receipts. If a particular item arrives without the expected instructions, don't pay for it until you receive them.

6. Ask the installer what parts are likely to wear out first in the equipment. Order spares now.

7. Be sure cabinets are installed in correct locations and are level. Have proper plumbing hookups been done?

8. Does the equipment work as anticipated? If you've chosen your supplier with care for his service capability and reliability, this is when it should pay off.

9. Check all drawers, slides, and other hardware for proper operation.

57
EXTRA TOUCHES

The ideas and accessories discussed in this chapter can make your office more comfortable, agreeable, or efficient without large outlays of money. Some of them will enhance your office by their beauty. Others will provide some convenience for your patients, which indicates that you're sensitive to their needs.

Although these are among the last items installed, they shouldn't be afterthoughts. Some of them may have to be planned for very early in the design stages. For instance, if you're thinking of having living plants in a part of the office where natural lighting will be inadequate, you'll have to make provision for enough artificial lighting to promote growth.

The principles that applied in the selection of your furniture, floor coverings, and wall coverings (see Chapter 37) should be carried over to the selection of your finishing touches. These can include:

1. Planters. Look for floor planters and hanging containers with a variety of graceful, interesting shapes and in colors that harmonize with other colors around them (Figures 57-1A, 1B, 1C).

2. Plants. Try to choose plants with smooth-edged—not saw-toothed—contours. Avoid those with jagged shapes or sharp spines, such as cacti. Incidentally, be sure that any live plants in your reception room are nonpoisonous if young children will be in that room at any time. The local poison control center can tell you what to avoid. For a complete discussion of plants for use in the office, see *The Office Gardener*, by Jacqueline Heriteau, New York: Hawthorn Books, 1977.

3. Wall hangings:

Diplomas and certificates. You've earned them, and you're proud of them. Display them tastefully in groupings, not as a hodge-podge. And be sure they hang straight.

Paintings. Leave your avant-garde tastes at home if you're fond of wild colors and jagged shapes. They don't belong in your office. They'll upset many

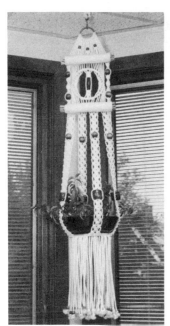
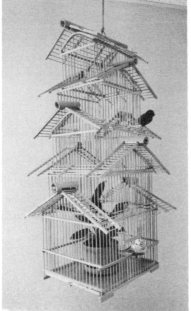
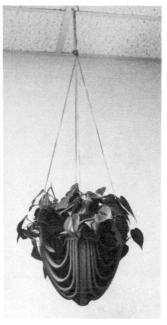

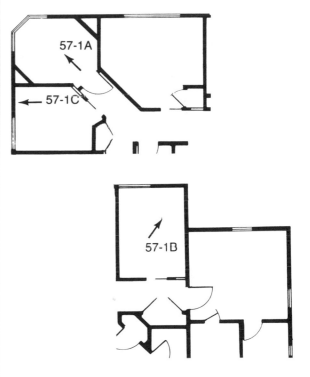

patients and will make them more anxious than they were before they arrived. Select artwork with pleasant themes and harmonizing colors.

Needlepoints, tapestries, and other wall-hung artwork. If you have a weaver or needlepointer in the family you may get some beautiful pieces for your walls (Figure 57-2).

Mirrors. Patients of both sexes like to check their appearance frequently, especially after a medical or dental visit.

Bulletin board. A bulletin board in the waiting room (Figure 57-2) with cartoons or items of interest is always fun. Place it where people reading it won't be in the traffic pattern and be sure to change its contents frequently.

4. Coat rack. The place where patients leave their coats in or near your reception room (Figure 57-3) should have a bar with sturdy hangers, a shelf for hats, a tray for overshoes, and a mirror. If you have many child patients, have

Figure 57-2. Reception room. This was the dining room of Victorian house, but was later used as living room after front half of building was destroyed by previous owners. Lovely black marble fireplace, dating from 1850s was a charred mess when we first saw it. Two marble experts worked for two days removing 125 years of soot. Bulletin board, made by a local frame shop, holds cartoons and topical items. Picture of sailboats, needlepointed by my wife, Marcia, shows scene typical of Tappan Zee, a wide expanse of the Hudson River near office.

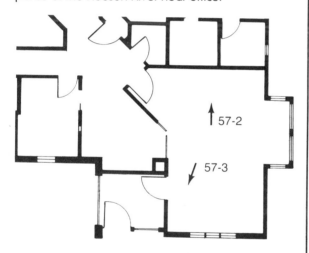

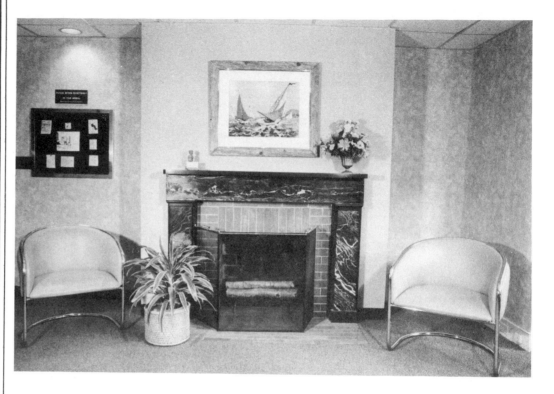

hooks for their coats low enough for them to reach. You'll prevent messy floors in other parts of the office if this area also has an umbrella stand and a floor mat for wiping snow-covered boots.

5. Treatment-room amenities. Your patient's clothing doesn't have to be draped on your cabinets, your operating stool, or the floor. In our dental-treatment rooms, a man can hang his jacket on a nearby hook (Figure 57-4A) placed where he can see it. Women appreciate the convenience of a hand-bag shelf (Figure 57-4B), which avoids putting the bag on the floor.

If you're a physician whose patients must undress, give some thought to the kind of dressing area you'd want if you were the patient. This means a chair or bench, curtains (down to ankle length) that close properly, a mirror, a bar or hook for hanging clothes, hangers (wood, not wire), and a comfortably sized and level shelf. The devices shown in Figures 57-3 and 57-4A and 4B can be modified and used in such a dressing area.

6. Magazine rack. A wall-mounted magazine rack (Figure 57-4C) in the reception room keeps magazines neat and off the chairs and floor. We found that some of the more popular magazines were disappearing regularly until we put them in plastic binders. People who are ready to pilfer a magazine for an interesting article or recipe seem to restrain themselves when the issues are in a binder. Consider small racks for magazines in treatment rooms, too, if patients will be left alone there for long periods.

Keep your magazines current. No monthly publication should be more than one month old. No weekly should be out for more than two weeks.

7. Clipboard. Your patients will find a clipboard in the reception room (Figure 57-4D) useful for filling out insurance forms and medical histories. Without it, they'll lean on magazines or chair arms. Ballpoint ink is impossible to remove from vinyl upholstery, so the clipboard will help your furniture last longer.

8. Plate glass identification. If you have any expanse of plate glass in the office, make it obvious that the glass is there. Signs, decals, or artificial flowers mounted on the glass will call attention to its presence (see Figures 41-4A and 4B). Before we did this, one of our patients—a lawyer, no less!—leaned over a counter to talk with our insurance clerk. Since the glass there was spotlessly clean, he didn't see it and wound up with a bump on his head. Fortunately, there were no serious sequelae, medical or legal.

9. Signs. Be sure that the lettering on all signs is large enough to be read easily, that the proportions of the sign are pleasing, and that the grammar and the spelling are correct.

Most of the signs in our office are white lettering on a chocolate-brown background. They harmonize with other colors in the office.

Since our building is set far back from the street, we wanted a sign that would clearly show our street number. Our original plan called for the installation of a custom-designed column near the street end of our driveway to display the number. When we received bids that were several times the amount we had budgeted, we decided something else had to be done.

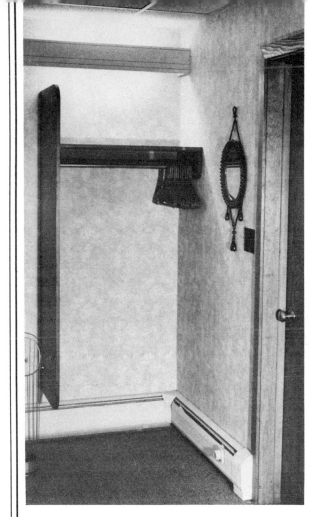

Figure 57-3. Patients' coat rack in reception room next to entry door. Architect's simple but functional design was built by cabinetmaker with plastic laminate that matches furniture. Shelf provides space for hats. Umbrella stand is at left. Small mirror is appreciated by patients. A small-scale version of this rack would be appropriate for the dressing area in a physician's examining room.

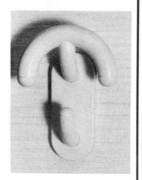

Our solution was to engage an artist who uses vivid colors and designs in her paintings. The sign she painted for us hangs just behind the plate-glass window next to our front door (Figure 57-5). Since the numbers are 12 inches high, they're easily seen from the street. The bright colors are a foretaste of the color scheme in the office.

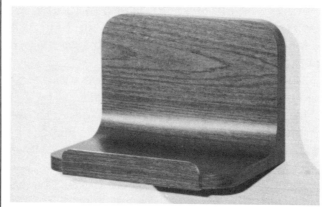

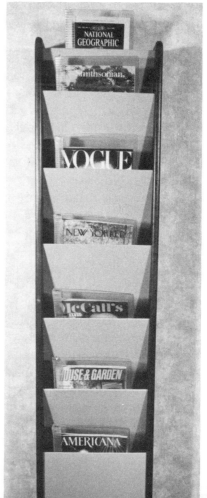

Figure 57-4A. Clothes hook. Each treatment room has one of these handy gadgets. Patient can hang jacket on lower hook or just drape it over the upper rounded portion. Available at houseware shops.

Figure 57-4B. Handbag shelf. Plastic laminate matches cabinet countertop. Front lip is aluminum angle bracket to which plastic laminate was cemented. If you use such a shelf, be sure it's hung level and within view of patient.

Figure 57-4C. Magazine rack. Wall-hung rack keeps magazines neat and off floor and furniture.

Figure 57-4D. Clipboard, hung on wall outside insurance secretary's desk, gives patients firm surface for filling out insurance forms.

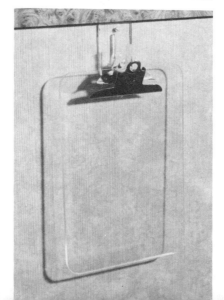

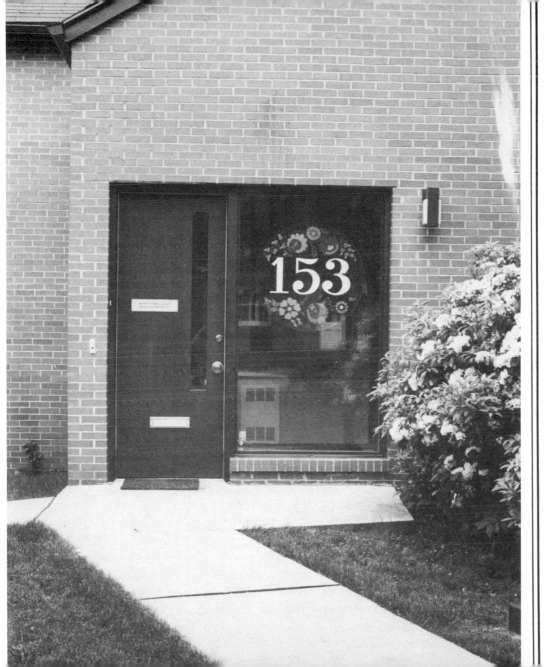

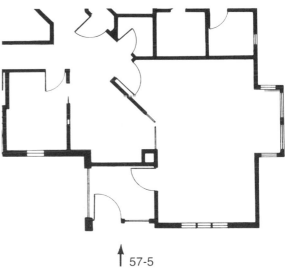

↑ 57-5

Figure 57-5. Office entry and sign. Foot-high white numbers are surrounded by bright yellow, red, orange, and blue flowers. Sign, painted by a local artist, is on clear plastic disk suspended behind double-glazed plate glass. Door opens into vestibule.

58

MOVING DAY

If you plan well for this day (see Chapter 54), you'll be prepared for almost anything.

Since we moved on a Monday, we arranged for the entire staff to be in on Saturday and Sunday. Each person was assigned to a particular area to pack. As each carton was filled, it was sealed shut with a strip of two-inch vinyl tape and labeled in large letters with its contents and its destination in the new office, for example: "Insurance forms—Sec'y office," or "Diplomas—Pvt. office."

The prepared identifying tags were attached to all pieces of furniture. Instrument and file cabinets that were to be moved with their contents still inside were taped shut after we were absolutely sure that nothing inside would rattle around and break.

On Monday morning, while the movers carried out the furniture and about 60 cartons, the equipment company's servicemen disconnected our old equipment and prepared it for the movers.

Since our new office was only a few blocks from the old one, the move itself took only a few minutes. We spent Monday afternoon and Tuesday unpacking and putting things away, while our equipment installation was going on. (Two treatment rooms of new equipment had been fully installed the week before.) We probably could have seen patients on Tuesday afternoon, but we gave ourselves that full day to sort things out and clean up.

Following are some tips that should help to make your move nontraumatic:

1. Arrange to have the new office swept and vacuumed just before moving day. This will prevent sharp objects—nails, screws, construction debris—from being ground into your floor coverings by the movers' boots and dollies.

2. Spread plastic runners or painters' drop cloths in heavily traversed areas, again to protect the floors. This is especially important in winter if sand or salt is likely to be tracked in.

3. Have plenty of cleaning supplies available, including bucket, sponge, rags, broom, dustpan, detergents, scouring powders, scrub brush, and a good vacuum cleaner. Prepare the office lavatories with soap, toilet paper, paper towels, and wastebaskets.

4. You'll need tools to put up chart racks, towel dispensers, mirrors, certificates, and pictures. We found these handy: hammer, screwdrivers, electric drill and bits, small stepladder, and assorted fasteners—picture hooks, hollow-wall anchors, and screws of different sizes. Sheet metal screws are usually best because they're threaded for their entire length.

5. If you're moving far enough away from your old office to require a new phone number, call the old number on moving day or the next morning. The intercept operator should come on the line to inform the caller of the change of phone number.

6. Call "Information" to find out if your new number is being given to callers.

7. If any item appears to have been damaged during the move, insist that the driver note on the bill that a claim is to be made for that particular article.

Even with all of these preparations, we still ran into some problems. A January snow and ice storm on the Friday before our move led to some anxiety about whether the movers and equipment people would get there on time. They did. Temporary difficulties with the heating system in the new office made the quick purchase of some electric heaters a necessity.

But all things considered, I think we did reasonably well, and we soon settled into the new surroundings with all systems functioning.

X
AFTERMATH

59
GETTING THE BUGS OUT

During the first few weeks in your new office (and building), expect that some things will go wrong. Leaks may develop in old or new equipment, doors will bind, and various things won't work. This early break-in period can be trying, but if you've done your planning wisely and selected your experts, your builder, and your suppliers with care, the problems aren't likely to be catastrophic.

Once again, a punch list is a must. Every time a drawer sticks, a switch feels loose, or a fixture won't stay put, write it down. Unless the problem is really major, you won't be able to get the builder back each time something goes wrong. But if you present him with a detailed list when he does come, you've got a reasonable chance of getting things done.

This is when you'll appreciate having that 10 percent retainage (holdback) provision—suggested in Chapter 35—in your contract. It should call for the final payment to be made 20 or 30 days after you move in.

During this period, identify as many of the problems as possible, because the builder will still be anxious about pleasing you. Once he's received that final payment, you'll have much less leverage. If he and his subcontractors are reliable, you'll get things done, but probably a little more slowly.

These first days are also the time to acquaint your staff with the workings of all your new equipment and how it is to be maintained, as well as with the details of special emergency procedures. Here are a few for you to consider:

1. Who is to do each necessary procedure if a patient becomes acutely ill in the office? Everyone ought to know how to turn on the oxygen and where the emergency drugs are kept.

2. Have you posted a list of emergency phone numbers at each phone? Include fire, police, hospital, and ambulance corps.

3. Do you and does everyone else in your office know how to free a child who's accidentally locked himself in a lavatory? Keep the key accessible.

4. Does everyone know how to turn the alarm system on and off? Someone who doesn't ordinarily come early or stay late may have to operate it one day. Also, your regular maintenance people will have to be taught how to turn it on and off.

5. Have you compiled a list of people to call if problems develop with equipment, plumbing, locks, appliances, office machines, or alarm systems?

6. Have you set up maintenance schedules? They are discussed in detail in Chapter 60. Do it now; later, it will be more difficult.

60
OFFICE AND BUILDING MAINTENANCE

Once your new office (and building) is completed, it makes good sense to safeguard your huge investment by a systematic maintenance program. If you introduce it promptly after moving in, it will be just one of many new procedures to which your staff will adapt. But if you wait weeks or months, your attempt to start these routines may meet resistance.

OFFICE MAINTENANCE

A good office-maintenance program needs these characteristics:

1. It should state in writing:

☐ what exactly is to be done: naming the equipment or other part of the office needing care and what care should consist of (follow the manufacturer's recommendations);

☐ when it is to be done: daily, weekly, monthly; and

☐ who is to do it: This assignment of responsibility is one of the most important features of a good program. Each office assistant should know which jobs are hers. We keep maintenance schedules posted in the office. As each job is done, the person who does it initials that part of the schedule. This immediately tells us if a job hasn't been done due to illness or vacation, for example. Then someone else is delegated to do it.

2. As much as possible, the program should be created by the staff, using volunteers if appropriate. Less pleasant jobs may have to be assigned and rotated among different staff members.

3. The jobs most likely to be overlooked are those to be done monthly or less frequently. A useful technique is to do them when some regularly scheduled event occurs. We've found that certain monthly tasks, like testing our alarm bells and changing over our central suction system from one pump to another (we alternate the use of them monthly), can be conveniently done on the day of our monthly lunchtime staff meeting. At this time, too, we change the setting on the clock switch that controls the outside lights (as the days shorten or lengthen).

Table 60-1 is a list of some maintenance jobs that should be done regularly. Add your own and delete the inappropriate items. Some of the jobs listed may be done by office staff or by outside individuals or companies.

You can get excellent material about maintenance from manufacturers and trade organizations. DuPont, for example, publishes a maintenance manual for carpets of DuPont nylon, Antron nylon, and Dacron polyester. Write to Carpet Maintenance Specialist, E.I. DuPont de Nemours and Co. Inc., Centre Road Building, Wilmington, Del. 19898. Another source of information is the Carpet and Rug Institute, Dalton, Ga. 30720.

The Armstrong Cork Company of Lancaster, Pa., publishes a sheet called "Maintenance Systems for Armstrong Commercial Floors" that describes the care of resilient floor covering. Other information on care of such flooring is available from the Resilient Floor Covering Institute, 1030 15th Street, N.W., Suite 350, Washington, D.C. 20005.

ENERGY CONSERVATION IN THE OFFICE

The reduction of energy consumption is as important in your office as in the management of a building. The following measures and those in Chapter 26 were suggested in a checklist developed by the Council on Dental Practice of the American Dental Association, published Sept. 17, 1979, in *ADA News*. They are reprinted by permission. (An additional list of conservation measures for a building can be found in Chapter 26.)

"Test windows and [outside] doors for air tightness.

"Close off empty rooms and adjust temperature.

TABLE 60-1

Office and equipment maintenance jobs

Letters in parentheses refer to the frequency with which these chores are done in our office:

D = Daily	SA = Semiannually
SW = Semiweekly	A = Annually
W = Weekly	PRN = As needed
M = Monthly	FMR = Following manufacturer's recommendations

General office maintenance

Cleaning:
- Dust (SW)
- Sweep (SW)
- Vacuum (SW)
- Polish (W)
- Spot removal (PRN)
- Empty trash containers (D)

Lavatories:
- Clean (SW)
- Replace paper supplies (PRN)
- Replace deodorant supplies (PRN)

Plants:
- Water (W or PRN)
- Trim and re-pot (PRN)

Remove and replace old magazines (W)

Clean, defrost refrigerator (M)

Wax floors (M)

Wash windows (PRN)

Shampoo carpets (SA)

Test alarm systems (M)

Inspect fire extinguishers (SA)

Change air-conditioner filters (A)

Change in-line water filter (A)

Change light bulbs (PRN)

continued

Professional equipment maintenance

Clean and lubricate hinged instruments before
    sterilizing (PRN)

Lubricate heavy equipment (FMR)

Flush and clean central suction lines (D)

Clean solids collected in central suction lines:

    in treatment rooms (W)

    at pump (M)

Autoclave:

    flush and change water (W)

    clean interior (M)

Change cold sterilizing solution (W)

Alternate use of:

    air compressors (M)

    suction pumps* (M)

*If your central suction unit requires a continuous flow of water, put a label on the valve that controls the office's water supply, with a warning written in large letters that says, "Do NOT close this valve until central suction unit is turned off." This will prevent the burn-out of the suction unit if water must be turned off for a plumbing repair.

"Dust or vacuum radiators frequently to promote heat flow.

"Adjust draperies throughout the day to let in or keep out heat or cold.

"Turn off lights, units, laboratory equipment, and electrical appliances when not in use."

BUILDING MAINTENANCE

Long before your building is occupied, you ought to start planning a maintenance program. The following checklist was developed for use in large commercial office buildings, but it contains many suggestions that are useful to owners of small professional buildings, too. It appeared in "Office Building Openings: A Checklist" by R.F. Muhlebach and F.E. Ryan, *Buildings*, December 1979, and is reprinted by permission.

☐ Negotiate maintenance contracts:

Cleaning

Landscaping

Security

Alarm/sprinkler system

Piped-in music

Elevator—construction contracts for elevator installations frequently include up to three months' maintenance.

☐ "Order tools and equipment for maintenance staff.

☐ "Hire building maintenance staff.

☐ "Test mechanical equipment with installers. This should be done prior to the building being turned over to [you].

☐ "Develop a preventive maintenance program (with building maintenance staff).

☐ "Meet with the landscaping and cleaning contractors to develop a preventive maintenance program.

☐ "Develop a form for use on building inspections. Form should list all items which need attention, what appropriate action is taken, and the date completed. These forms should be kept on file.

☐ "Prior to the first tenant move-in, [have] building common areas pre-cleaned and tenant suites pre-cleaned.

- [ ] "Meet with the cleaning contractor to develop a program to conserve energy by cleaning efficiently.
- [ ] "[All owner-tenants and maintenance staff] should walk [through] the building to become familiar with all common areas, especially building exits and use of fire extinguishers. They should be familiar with the location of mechanical equipment, shut-off valves, and circuit breakers, and know where each exit door leads.
- [ ] "Consider installing temporary carpet in elevators and lobby during tenant construction phase, when the building [shell] is occupied.
- [ ] "Develop a building keying system.
- [ ] "Keep on file all building plans, including plans for the mechanical and electrical systems.
- [ ] "Walk the building with police and fire departments to familiarize them with the building and its operation.
- [ ] "Estabish emergency procedures for bomb threats, fire, and other potential disasters.
- [ ] "Develop a list of all the general contractor's subcontractors who worked on the building. Include their telephone numbers and after-hours emergency telephone numbers.
- [ ] "Develop a list of all contractors who will work on the building, including their telephone numbers and emergency after-hours telephone numbers. Also, include the home telephone numbers of all building personnel [and owner-tenants].
- [ ] "Develop a list of all contacts and their telephone numbers for all utility companies servicing the building. Include the police, fire, building, and health departments.
- [ ] "Obtain copies of all construction contracts for future reference and warranty.
- [ ] "Obtain all warranties.
- [ ] "Review energy conservation and walk [through] the building with the utility company representatives for their conservation suggestions.
- [ ] "Coordinate the placement of the building's insurance with the phasing out of the construction insurance.
- [ ] "Develop a security system for the building."

If your building is too small to warrant a full-time maintenance person—and that's likely—you'll have to find a local handyman to do many of the necessary jobs. Reliability and availability are the most important attributes to look for. You won't want to be called from a patient to unstop a toilet or to shovel snow yourself.

XI
FINAL NOTES

61

HELPFUL
GADGETS
AND SYSTEMS

Our office has a number of devices and systems that you may find useful. I'm including in this chapter those that are a little out of the ordinary. You can build low-voltage circuits for them yourself, if your home workshop has metalworking tools. Other possible sources are a local electronics hobbyist, an electrician, or the installers of your burglar alarm, intercom, or telephone equipment.

WATER ALARM

Your office may have a basement or utility area that is not visited on a daily basis. In such a location, water that is leaking from a boiler, a water heater, or other equipment can accumulate undetected. The simple "aspirin alarm" show in Figures 61-1A and 1B will alert you to the presence of a leak almost as soon as it occurs.

ANNUNCIATOR

Depending on your office layout, you may want a system that informs you or a staff member in a remote part of the office that someone has entered or left the reception room. Such systems are available at electrical supply outlets. They consist of a floor mat or "electric eye" sensor that sounds a chime when activated. We use a modification of the same idea.

In the jamb of our front door we have a normally closed (NC) pushbutton, the type often used in burglar-alarm systems. This is pressed in (breaking the circuit) when the door closes and released (completing the circuit) when the door opens. It's connected in a simple series circuit to a 12-volt DC power supply and to a signal light in the sterilization area (see Figure 42-3B). On those occasions when only one assistant is working, the light with its accompanying "click" alerts her to the opening of the front door. Additional lights and/or audible signals can be placed anywhere in the office.

ASSISTANT-CALL SYSTEM

We didn't need one of the multilight silent intercoms described in Chapter 29, but we wanted a method of calling an assistant to a specific room. A homemade signal system was the result.

When the call button is pressed In a treatment room or in the private office, a buzzer sounds in the sterilization alcove. A light goes on in the hall outside the room where the assistant is needed. The assistant, alerted by the buzzer, looks down the hall for the lit signal lamp (a bright green, 12-volt lamp shown in Figure 61-2; the circuit arrangement is shown in Figure 61-3; Figure 61-4 shows how the components were mounted) As she enters the room, she presses the reset button to turn off the light. In many ways, the system operates like a nurse-call system in a hospital.

The relays used throughout this system are electromechanical devices. They depend on the up-and-down movement of an armature in response to the activation of the relay's coil. With time, all such devices can fail. For this reason, the relays selected are sealed in plastic enclosures. Each plugs into a matching socket. If a relay fails, it's a simple matter to unplug it and install a new one. If you're wondering why 12-volt DC relays were used, it's because 12-volt power supplies are inexpensive and easy to find and because I've heard that DC relays seem to last longer than the AC type.

A few general comments about building and installing any of these low-voltage systems:

1. Plan them far in advance of installation. You'll need time to order essential parts.

2. If you get a silent intercom, some of the functions of my systems will be included in the intercom's light arrangements, or you may be able to have them installed for an extra charge.

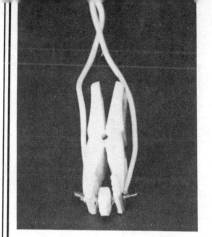

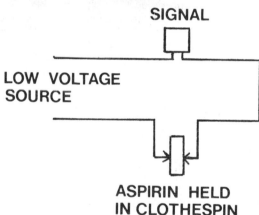

SIGNAL

LOW VOLTAGE
SOURCE

ASPIRIN HELD
IN CLOTHESPIN

Figure 61-1A. Aspirin alarm. Aspirin tablet is held in spring clothespin that has been modified with small bolts. Homemade device is placed on floor in areas where undetected water leakage is possible. If leak occurs, tablet dissolves and jaws come together, closing circuit and sounding alarm.

Figure 61-1B. Aspirin-alarm circuit. System works like a doorbell. When aspirin dissolves in water, contacts close and a simple series circuit sounds the alarm. You can use any low voltage, AC or DC. Just be sure that your signal works on the same voltage.

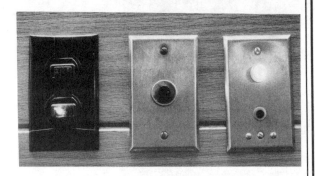

Figure 61-2. Switches and signals. From left: On-off switch and pilot light for X-ray machine, exposure push-button switch for X-ray, and assistant call signal lamp. This lamp stays lit until assistant pushes button.

Figure 61-3. Assistant call signal circuit. *Latching* action of DPDT relay keeps lamp lit after button (A_1/A_2) is pressed. A_1 and A_2 are parts of one switch, a double-pole, single throw (DPST), normally open, momentary pushbutton switch. Pressing this button activates both circuits. A_2 makes the buzzer sound and stops when button is released. At the same time, closing A_1 energizes the coil of DPDT relay. The two armature contacts, B and C, are pulled down. When B is down, terminals 1 and 2 are connected, completing the latching circuit. This bypasses A_1 and keeps the relay's coil energized after A_1 is released. When C is down, it completes the signal-lamp circuit through terminals 4 and 5. The lamp stays lit while the coil is energized. When the normally closed reset button is pressed, the latching circuit is broken, armature springs up, and lamp goes off.

If you can't find DPST pushbutton switches or if your existing equipment has single-pole call buttons, you can still use this system. You'll need a second DPDT relay. Your single-pole pushbutton can activate that relay's coil. One set of armature contacts can sound the buzzer (replacing A_2); the other set can activate the original relay's coil (replacing A_1).

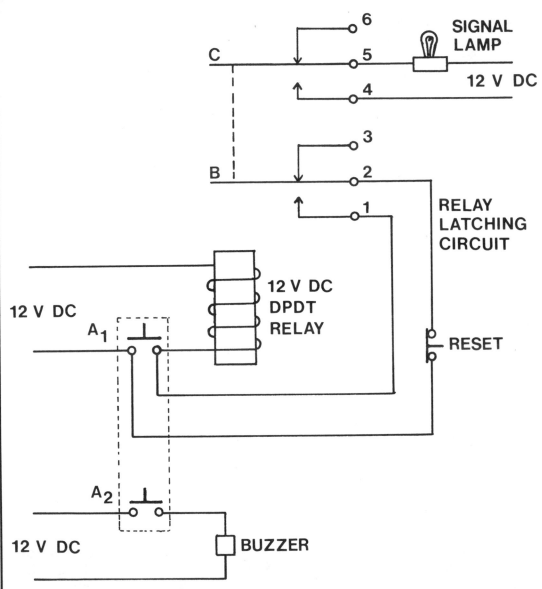

3. You'll find some of the necessary parts in a local electronics store. For the relays and special switches, you may have to search harder. The major mail-order electronics suppliers are good sources.

4. I've found that the best way to install custom-made volume controls and signal lights is this: At a local electrical supply house buy blank, brushed, stainless-steel wall plates. Such plates are sturdy and durable. They look as if they belong in a professional office, especially if you're careful to locate the mounted lamps or switches neatly and symmetrically (see Figure 61-2). Ask for either the *one gang* ($2\frac{3}{4}'' \times 4\frac{1}{2}''$) or *two gang* ($4\frac{1}{2}'' \times 4\frac{1}{2}''$) size, depending on what you intend to mount on them. Buy the corresponding plaster rings, too, for installation during the rough-in stage. When you drill holes in the wall plates, be careful not to mar the brushed finish.

5. Be prepared with plenty of 18/2 wire (solid or stranded) and allow lots of time for the rough-in stage. If there are places in the office for which you may need a volume control or signal lamp in the future, but not now, do this: Run the wires to that location and install a plaster ring. When the walls are closed, screw a blank stainless-steel wall plate to the plaster ring. The wires hidden in the wall will be accessible whenever you need them.

6. Buy spares now of parts that can burn out or break, such as lamps or relays.

7. Label all your low-voltage wires with paper tags (see Figure 49-1J) to avoid confusion later.

8. Draw circuit diagrams and describe each homemade system in writing. It may need repair in your absence.

HELPFUL GADGETS

Figures 61-5A and 5B show a pair of devices we have found useful. The hanger lets you suspend planters from any part of a dropped ceiling's grid. The chart rack is excellent if you can't find a ready made holder for patient records.

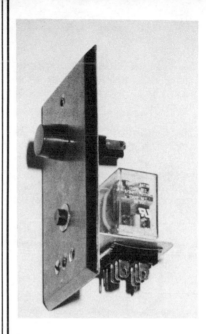

Figure 61-4. Side view of assistant call signal shows mounting of components before wires are connected. Bracket with cutout for relay socket is made of sheet metal and is attached to wall plate by machine screws and nuts.

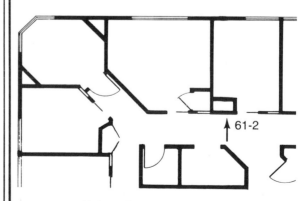

61-2

Figure 61-5A. Hanger for use with dropped ceiling. This useful two-piece gadget clips to either side of ceiling grid and lets you suspend a hanging plant anywhere in office.

Figure 61-5B. Custom-made chart rack holds one day's charts for one doctor. Several of them were made by a local plastics fabricator of one-quarter-inch white acrylic plastic. Dimensions: 11½" W × 11"H (at rear). Interior opening: 4¼" front to back. List of patients on front is held by clip with soft wax on back, which sticks to plastic.

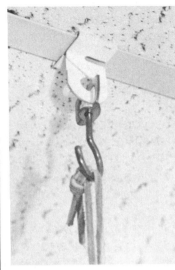

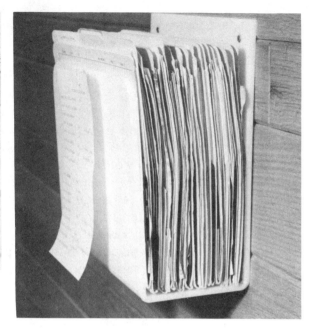

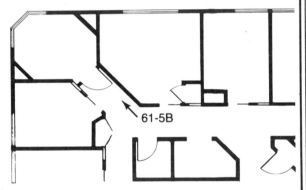

62

OUR RENOVATION OF AN OLD BUILDING

During the summer of 1976 my partner, Mike Savin, and I decided that the time had come to find a larger office for our periodontal practice. We wanted to stay in or near the same community, but we quickly found that no suitable rental space was available or about to be built. We thought seriously about putting up our own building, but the most attractive possibility seemed to be the conversion of an old house to an office.

Our community is a lovely old Hudson Valley village. The first settlers arrived in the 17th century, and there are many well-cared-for homes that are more than 100 years old. Along Broadway, which runs parallel to the river, some of the old houses had been renovated for use as professional offices. That's what we wanted to do, too.

In late October, our local insurance agent, who is also a real-estate broker, told us of an old house that had just come on the market. It had been the home of an elderly widower who had died the year before. The building was in a stable part of town a few blocks from our old office. Since it was only three blocks from the hospital, it had good potential for sale to a physicians' group at some time in the future. This made the single-office aspect less of an investment risk.

As soon as we saw the property, we felt it was what we were looking for. The house was 70 feet back from the street on a half-acre site with some lovely old trees. Split-rail fences in disrepair separated it from the properties on either side (Figure 62-1).

The building itself was unimpressive. Its exterior was partly brick and partly wood-siding. The floor plan didn't appear to make sense (see Figure 19-1).

Figure 62-1. The old house as it looked when we bought it in 1976. Original Victorian structure was built in mid-19th century. It had been mutilated by previous owners in 1950s, probably to save on taxes. They cut off and discarded front half of building, then put up brick veneer. We changed facade and salvaged most of the landscaping, including taxus and mountain laurel shrubs near front entry and the huge hydrangea at left.

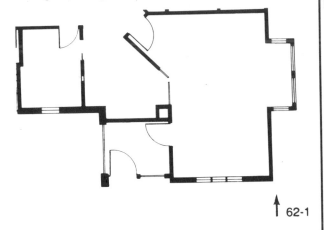

↑ 62-1

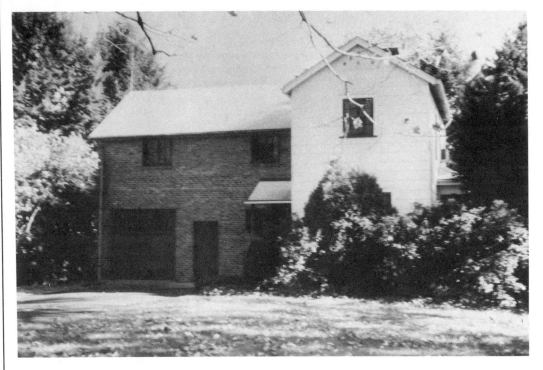

There was one large room, apparently the living room, with a sooty fireplace, a kitchen, a bath, and a small room at the rear, which was last used as a bedroom. Also on the lower level was a one-car garage. Upstairs were two spacious bedrooms and a bath. Half the house had a basement under it. The rest was built on a slab.

The rooms on the first floor were arranged in a peculiar way, and there was no dining room. This was most unusual for a Victorian house. Much of the building looked at least 100 years old. We learned later that it was built in the 1850s.

Another puzzler was why the house was set so far back from the sidewalk when all of its neighbors' front doors were close to the street. And why was the house so much smaller than those nearby? Its first-floor area, including the garage, was only about 1,000 square feet.

The answer to these mysteries came later from a neighbor: The original house was a big rambling Victorian that was as close to the street as any of its neighbors. In the 1950s the owners decided that the house was too big for them; they had a builder literally chop away and cart off the whole front half of the building and then put up a brick veneer wall to close the wound in the part that remained.

This explained, too, why the room arrangement was strange. We were looking at half a house. These rooms had been only the back section of the original building. What we thought was the living room was the original dining room. The huge living room or parlor and some rooms upstairs were in the section that was demolished. Later, when the parking area was being graded, we encountered the foundation of the front half of the original building.

Our first step was to call Bill Kohn. William Eli Kohn, A.I.A., was the architect who had designed my home 12 years earlier, and he had helped me convert my original office to a more efficient floor plan. I knew that he was experienced in office design and that Mike and I could work with him.

Bill's impression, after looking over the house, was that it was structurally sound, but we'd have to add to it to get the office size we needed—about 2,000 square feet. He had an engineer review the mechanical systems. The report included the opinions that the gas-fired, hot-water boiler might be usable and that the electrical wiring would have to be completely replaced. We also learned that there was no sign of termites around the foundation.

While these inspections were going on, we checked on the zoning. The neighborhood was zoned for one- and two-family residences, but there were enough houses converted to offices within the space of a few blocks nearby to provide us with ample precedents for a variance.

The amount asked for the property was reasonable, and after a short period of negotiation we settled on a price. A contract was drawn up that stipulated that the sale would be final if, and only if, we were able to obtain the necessary zoning variance. This would be permission to use the lower floor for professional offices and the upper story for an apartment.

The zoning hearing was held about six weeks later, in late December. Bill, after many meetings with us, was able to bring along some preliminary plans and a cardboard model of what the finished structure would probably look like. This was to show the zoning board and any neighbors present at the hearing that we would be maintaining the character of the neighborhood and improving the property.

There was no opposition to our petition for a variance, but at the request of our next-door neighbor, the proposed on-site parking was reduced from 10 cars to seven. Since street parking is permitted, this has not created a hardship.

Once the zoning hurdle was cleared, the *closing* or final transfer of the land and building to us could take place. Interestingly, a survey showed that the property was not quite as large as it had been originally represented to be. As a result, we were able to negotiate a proportionate decrease in the price.

Planning and design now went full speed ahead. By late April 1977, a final set of plans and specs were distributed to several local builders. All of the bids were higher than we'd hoped for, but one of them was close enough so that after Bill Kohn made some design modifications and some further negotiation occurred, we were able to agree on a lump-sum contract for the job.

The bidding, redesign, negotiation, and contract review all took another six weeks, until early June. The builders started work on June 22, 1977. Seven months later, on January 23, 1978, we moved in. This was 15 months after we first saw the property, not an unusual time span. Figure 62-2 shows the building as it looks today. Figure 19-4 is the final floor plan.

In retrospect, our renovation plus new construction went smoothly enough, although we had our share of delays, problems, and extra costs:

1. The existing gas-fired, 15-year-old boiler was replaced with a new one when it became apparent that since all new pipes, valves, and controls had to be installed anyway for the hot-water heating system, the savings we'd gain by keeping the old boiler just weren't worth risking a breakdown (extra cost: $500). By the way, the *new* boiler needed repairs during its first year!

2. The new wing was located next to the portion of the old house that was built on a slab. We didn't know until the excavation was done just how deep this part of the old foundation went. When we found that it didn't go down

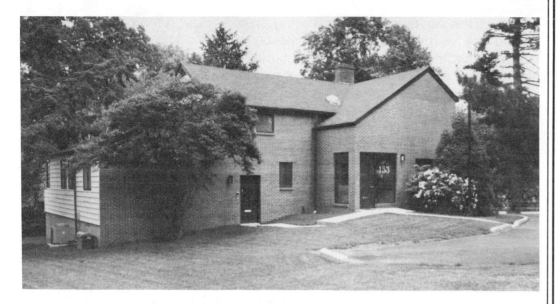

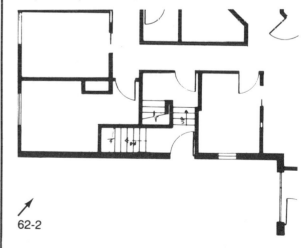

62-2

as far as our new basement, the builders had to underpin it with cement blocks. These had the effect of lowering the old foundation to the new level (extra cost: $1,100).

3. The windows for the new wing of the building were delivered about six weeks late. This delayed much of the interior work, since the wing couldn't be closed in until the windows were installed.

4. With the increased cost of energy, we wanted our building to be well insulated. While construction was going on, we decided to add more attic insulation. We also added a layer of Styrofoam insulation to the outer surface of the entire building before the outer skin of vinyl siding and brick veneer were installed (extra cost: $1,800). This extra work has since proved its value in fuel costs, which are lower than anticipated.

Our old building had some pleasant surprises for us, too. The messy, charred fireplace in the large front room, which became our reception room, turned into a source of pride after two marble experts spent a weekend restoring and polishing its lovely veined black marble surfaces (see Figure 57-2).

One of the advantages of converting an old house is the possibility of obtaining one or more apartments in the building in addition to the office. By adding a kitchen upstairs, we were able to create a comfortable, one-bedroom apartment. The rent it brings in helps the building's cash flow, while the presence of the tenant at night and on weekends helps to reduce our security problems.

It's difficult to assign costs per square foot when renovation is combined with new construction because much of the work involves both areas. The following figures for our job are approximations based on our architect's calculations:

☐ new construction: $53 per square foot (includes new wing, tie-in of new wing to old building, site work, and new mechanical systems for the whole building);

☐ construction of new basement storage area: $10 per square foot;

☐ renovation of old portion of first floor: $22 per square foot; and

☐ renovation of second-floor apartment: $12 per square foot.

Note that these figures include architectural and engineering fees, but they don't include the cost of the land or the old building. Also, these costs were incurred in 1977-78 and for this particular building. Every old building has its own problems and costs.

Would we do it again? Absolutely! As owners and as landlords we've had problems that we didn't have when we were leasing an office. But our satisfaction with our own building and office far outweighs these annoyances. The ideas described in this book worked effectively for us. I hope they work as well for you.

INDEX

Withdrawal from partnership, 62-63
Work letter, 35

X
X-ray
    electrical needs, 125
    legal requirements, 147, 148
    radiation physicists, 147, 240
    shielding, 17, 147-148
    switches, 127
    view box, 101

Z
Zones—office, 91, 92, 93, 95, 96, 149
Zoning, 18, 69-73
    architect and, 24, 70, 71, 72, 300
    building inspector and, 70, 71
    change of zone, 72
    history, 69
    home-office, 10, 44
    lawyer and, 20
    map, 65
    master plans, 69
    new building, 65
    ordinances, 69-70
    parking, 39, 70
    planning board, 71
    professional offices, 4, 70
    professional practice, 32, 39
    renovating old building, 9, 39, 299
    single-office building, 12
    site plan, 70-71
    site plan review, 71
    variances. See Zoning variances
Zoning ordinance, 69-72
    variances. See Zoning variances
    zoning board of appeals, 72
Zoning variances, 39, 41, 65, 72-73, 299